"An intelligent and accessible account of our current understanding of the complex interactions of biology, environment, and socio-economics in the etiology of obesity—arguably the most consequential long-term medical issue confronting the United States. Ahima—a widely admired physician-scientist—has studied this problem from many perspectives and is familiar with the broad range of relevant factors and their relationships. He encourages individuals with obesity through an emphasis on the biological basis for these problems and he offers scientific and public policy contexts for their ultimate solution. Such knowledge and awareness constitute important counterforces to persistent inclinations to blame individuals for this condition. Jargon-free and even-handed, the book will be useful to lay individuals as well as students and researchers as an excellent introduction to this very important problem."

—Rudolph L. Leibel, MD,
Christopher J. Murphy Memorial Professor of Diabetes Research,
Head, Division of Molecular Genetics, Columbia University

T0130777

"An appealing, easy-to-read, and balanced discussion of the disease of obesity, the drivers that influence it, and what can be done about it. The reader will come away with a much more informed view of obesity and a deeper understanding of the struggle faced by those suffering from it."

— Catherine Kotz, PhD, President, The Obesity Society; Professor, University of Minnesota; and Associate Director of Research (GRECC), Minneapolis VA Medical Center

"Dr. Ahima provides a rich, descriptive reading experience from the lab to the clinic and finally the food and built environment, shedding light on the complexities of obesity. His experience shines through in this update on treatment approaches and helpful strategies for those dealing with the chronic disease of obesity."

— Kelly C. Allison, PhD, Director, Center for Weight and Eating Disorders, and Professor, Department of Psychiatry, Perelman School of Medicine, University of Pennsylvania

Can the Obesity Crisis Be Reversed?

JOHNS HOPKINS
WAVELENGTHS

In classrooms, field stations, and laboratories in Baltimore and around the world, the Bloomberg Distinguished Professors of Johns Hopkins University are opening the boundaries of our understanding on many of the world's most complex challenges. The Johns Hopkins Wavelengths series brings readers inside their stories, presenting the pioneering discoveries and innovations that benefit people in their neighborhoods and across the globe in artificial intelligence, cancer research, food systems, health equity, planetary science, science diplomacy, and other critical areas of study. Through these compelling narratives, their insights will spark conversations from dorm rooms to dining rooms to boardrooms.

This print and digital media program is a partnership between the Johns Hopkins University Press and the University's Office of Research. Team members include:

Consultant Editor: Sarah Olson

Senior Acquisitions Editor: Matthew McAdam

Copyeditor: Charles Dibble

Art Director: Martha Sewall

Series Designer: Matthew Cole

Production Supervisor: Jennifer Paulson

Program Manager: Anna Marlis Burgard

JHUP Director and Publisher: Barbara Kline Pope

Office of Research Executive Director for Research: Julie Messersmith

Can the Obesity Crisis Be Reversed?

REXFORD S. AHIMA, MD, PhD

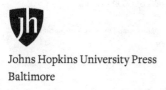

Johns Hopkins University Press
Baltimore

© 2021 Johns Hopkins University Press
All rights reserved. Published 2021
Printed in the United States of America on acid-free paper
9 8 7 6 5 4 3 2 1

Johns Hopkins University Press
2715 North Charles Street
Baltimore, Maryland 21218-4363
www.press.jhu.edu

Library of Congress Cataloging-in-Publication Data

Names: Ahima, Rexford S., author.
Title: Can the obesity crisis be reversed? / Rexford S. Ahima, MD, PhD.
Description: Baltimore : Johns Hopkins University Press, 2021. |
  Series: Johns Hopkins wavelengths | Includes bibliographical references
  and index.
Identifiers: LCCN 2021012208 | ISBN 9781421442716 (paperback) | ISBN
  9781421442723 (ebook) | ISBN 9781421442730 (ebook o)
Subjects: LCSH: Obesity. | Obesity—Treatment.
Classification: LCC RC628 .A354 2021 | DDC 362.1963/98—dc23
LC record available at https://lccn.loc.gov/2021012208

A catalog record for this book is available from the British Library.

*Special discounts are available for bulk purchases of this book. For more information,
please contact Special Sales at specialsales@jh.edu.*

Contents

Preface

ALTHOUGH I'VE SPENT MOST OF MY ADULT LIFE studying and practicing medicine, I fell into the study and treatment of obesity largely through circumstance. I was born and raised in Ghana, West Africa, where the education system is similar to the British system. In secondary (high) school, students are guided into choosing careers in the arts, sciences, or business. I attended the Accra Academy, in the capital city of Accra, where I excelled in the sciences and mathematics as well as music, art, and debate—the last of which probably helped shape my later propensity to question dogma and search for fresh ideas. In addition to speaking several native languages, we were all proficient in English, the national language of Ghana. Moreover, I studied French for three years and German for five years. All of these languages aided my studies and my career.

My mother worked for some years in nursing, which offered insights into the health profession and its impact on society. My father worked as an accountant in the civil service, and I may have gotten my knack for data and good recordkeeping from him. My brother enjoyed sports, which sharpened our competitiveness and provided a mutual escape from the monotony of schoolwork. I have very fond memories of growing up within an extended family in the sunny climate of Accra with its tropical rains, sports (soccer and track), great food, sandy beaches, and other lovely places.

After completing advanced science courses in high school and taking national examinations, I was admitted to the University of Ghana Medical School. The curriculum started with the basic sciences—anatomy, biochemistry, physiology, microbiology, pathology, and pharmacology—which offered lectures and laboratory work to establish a foundation for subsequent clinical training. I understood the connection between basic science and the illnesses afflicting people, such as infectious diseases, diabetes, heart diseases, and cancer. I did not, however, fully appreciate the importance of scientific research to the practice of medicine. Why did I need to know about research in order to prescribe a drug?

Fortunately, the dean of my medical school, Fred Nii Lomotey Engmann, had a different perspective. He had trained at the University of Cambridge, England, where medical students are required to spend a year focused on research (in what is known as an intercalated BSc degree) as part of their medical education. Professor Engmann decided to train Ghanaian students using the same kind of approach. As a result, he chose four students, myself included, to pursue an intercalated BSc training at the Middlesex Hospital Medical School of the University of London. It was a very successful program; out of my class of 20 students, 15 went on to receive PhDs in biomedical sciences.

That was how I found myself studying under the mentorship of R. Peter Gould at the Middlesex Hospital Medical School in 1980–81. Peter was the dean of students and a visionary in the fields of endocrinology and developmental biology. He said to me, "Rex, as a physician you'll have a very good life, you'll take care of hundreds of thousands of patients, maybe more, and they'll be very grateful. But if you want to have a huge impact, beyond what you can do personally, biomedical research gives you that option. In addition to helping your patients, the knowledge you gain can be helpful to other people, even after you're gone." Peter was a father figure—very kind and direct in his manner. He assembled an esteemed team of academicians to teach us and serve as role models, among them, Peter Campbell, Lewis Wolpert, John Tait, and Sylvia Tait at the Middlesex Hospital Medical School, and Ruth Bellairs at University College London. Peter gave me full access to an electron microscope and other sophisticated research technologies as I began doing my dissertation research on the development of the adrenal cortex—the endocrine gland right above the kidneys that synthesizes and secretes steroid hormones involved in the regulation of blood pressure and stress responses.

One highlight of my BSc training was presenting my research on the adrenal cortex at a meeting of the Anatomical Society of Great Britain and Ireland held in Sheffield, England. I was a bit nervous, but I remember Peter telling me with a broad smile, "Rex, you know your research better than me or anyone else in this audience. Your job is to teach us what you have done." That was his way of saying "Go get 'em!" Peter was a superb mentor and role model. We spent time with his family in Whitstable (three miles from Canterbury) and toured many towns in the English countryside. We traveled to Oxford and Cambridge to compare the universities with the sprawling University of London campus. In many ways, Peter regarded me as his peer rather than as his student. He challenged me to reach higher and become the best I could be. My BSc training in endocrinology taught me how hormones impact the body in many complex ways—during development, as part of normal organ function-ing, and in diseases. I was especially excited about being able to design specific studies using mouse models and electron microscopy to address fundamental mechanisms underlying endocrine and metabolic diseases, which affect more than 50 percent of the population.

Peter and I stayed in touch when I returned to Ghana to complete my clinical training and licensure. He encouraged me to apply to American programs for PhD training, saying that the United States offered the best opportunities for biomedical research. As a result, in 1988, I came to the United States to com-plete a PhD at Tulane University in New Orleans. Peter was right. Although the medical school systems in Ghana and the United Kingdom have many positive aspects, there's no doubt in my mind that the graduate education system in the United States tends to be more creative, which is why so many foreign students come here for graduate school and postdoctoral fellowships. My story is typical for generations of immigrant scientists who come to the United States to pursue their dreams. If the United States wants to remain a leader in science and medicine, it needs to continue to welcome students from abroad and provide them with opportunities to stay in this country.

Based on my background in adrenal research, I chose to work with Richard Harlan, an expert on the links between the endocrine system and the brain. In the 1970s, studies by Bruce McEwen, Donald Pfaff, and others at the Rockefeller University in New York City had offered new insights into how peripheral hormones synthesized elsewhere in the body acted in the brain to influence stress, memory, and complex behaviors. We studied this process for stress, mapped receptors in the brain for the steroid molecules known as glucocorticoids, and devised techniques to investigate gene expression in the brain. It was a highly productive period as we created new knowledge and opened frontiers for other researchers.

After finishing my PhD at Tulane in 1992, I completed my three-year internship and residency training in internal medicine at the Albert Einstein College of Medicine, Jack D. Weiler Hospital, and Jacobi Medical Center in the Bronx. From there, I went on to complete my clinical and research fellowship training in endocrinology, diabetes, and metabolism at the Beth Israel Deaconess Medical Center and at the Harvard Medical School in Boston. Although the focus of my work in all these places was the practice of medicine, I was fortunate to always be working with people who encouraged me to combine medicine and research, just as my previous mentors had done.

Then, in 1995, I got a lucky break. Scientists had long considered adipose tissue—otherwise known as body fat—to be an inactive tissue that stores the body's energy. However, previous studies had suggested that energy storage in adipose tissue was regulated by factors linking it to the brain. In the 1970s, Douglas Coleman, a Canadian working at the Jackson Laboratories in Bar Harbor, Maine, demonstrated that an unknown blood-borne factor was responsible for causing obesity in a genetic strain of mice known as ob/ob. He conducted cross-circulation experiments showing that the ob/ob mice lacked a hormone that suppressed feeding, while another strain, known as db/db mice, lacked the receptor mechanism capable of sensing this "obesity hormone." However, the source of the hormone and its tissue targets were unknown.

More than 20 years later, in 1994, Jeffrey M. Friedman at the Rockefeller University was finally able to prove the existence of a hormone, which he named leptin, that is secreted by fat tissue and plays a pivotal role in appetite and energy regulation. This discovery reversed long-held beliefs about the function of adipose tissue in the body. With the discovery of leptin, scientists quickly realized that body fat communicates with the brain and other organs not only through leptin but through many other peptide hormones (known as adipokines) to control energy balance, weight, and appetite. This discovery, which was my introduction to the study of obesity, was tremendously exciting.

In 1995, after completing my training in internal medicine, I embarked on a research fellowship at the Beth Israel Deaconess Medical Center in Boston with Jeffrey S. Flier, who later became the dean of the Harvard Medical School. Jeff and I hit it off right away. His background was in diabetes and obesity, while my background was in neuroendocrinology, so we could use our knowledge and skills to connect the hormonal interactions of the brain and peripheral organs. For three years, Jeff and I spent a lot of time trying to understand the functions of leptin. Among our seminal discoveries was that a fall in leptin during fasting suppressed thyroid and reproductive hormones and stimulated the stress response. We also studied leptin's role in the timing of puberty and brain development. In collaboration with colleagues at Harvard and elsewhere, we delineated the signaling pathways for leptin in the hypothalamus and other brain regions. Jeff is a master motivator, sharp thinker, and overall great personality. We've been friends for 25 years and counting!

My experience in Boston catalyzed my commitment to biomedical research. I was in the right place at the right time in an exciting field in which new discoveries were constantly being made. The discovery of leptin opened the way for me to ask questions regarding the molecular pathways underlying obesity, diabetes, and related diseases and to study how these pathways might be related to potential therapies.

After completing my fellowship with Jeff and spending another year as an instructor in medicine at the Beth Israel Deaconess Medical Center and Harvard Medical School, I was recruited by the University of Pennsylvania as an assistant professor in 1999. Research in my laboratory, mostly using mice as subjects, focused on understanding the molecular pathways connecting obesity with diabetes and related diseases. For example, in addition to leptin, I began studying two other major hormones related to energy balance called adiponectin and resistin. In part to attract other investigators to obesity, diabetes, and metabolism research, I founded and directed the Penn Mouse Metabolic Phenotyping Core. I also started a joint clinic with internists and specialists in cardiovascular medicine to provide comprehensive and integrated care for people with obesity, diabetes, and heart disease. This approach, which was based on understanding that obesity and diabetes affect multiple systems and require multiple care providers, was embraced by patients and providers.

I subsequently became the founder and director of Penn Metabolic Medicine, a multidisciplinary program for obesity and metabolic syndrome that links endocrinology, cardiovascular medicine, hepatology, bariatric surgery, and sleep medicine. I became associate director of the Institute for Diabetes, Obesity and Metabolism and was elected to the American Society for Clinical Investigation, the Association of American Physicians, the American Association for the Advancement of Science, the

American College of Physicians, and the Obesity Society. My 16 years at Penn were a wonderful time that gave me the opportunity to lead basic research in my laboratory as well as to create partnerships for advancing discovery, patient care, and education.

However, I also understood that the problems of obesity, diabetes, and related diseases require collaborative and advocacy efforts that go beyond the resources of a school of medicine. Therefore, in 2016, I accepted an offer to move to Johns Hopkins University as Bloomberg Distinguished Professor of Diabetes, professor of Medicine, Public Health and Nursing, and director of the Division of Endocrinology, Diabetes, and Metabolism. Here, I have been continuing my research into how adipokines act on the brain and other organs to control feeding, energy expenditure, and glucose and lipid metabolism. I have recruited new faculty and have forged collaborations across the university to conduct laboratory, clinical, and population studies that provide new insights into the causes, prevention, and treatment of obesity, diabetes, fatty liver, and cardiovascular disease. As the leader of the Johns Hopkins Diabetes Initiative, I work closely with colleagues across the Schools of Medicine, Public Health, and Nursing to promote basic, clinical, and population research and to translate new discoveries into diagnostic tools for the prevention and treatment of diabetes. I was especially proud to be elected to the National Academy of Medicine in 2020, since this organization has been a major advocate of the kinds of crossdisciplinary work that my position at Johns Hopkins has enabled me to do.

Since I began studying the neuroendocrinology of weight gain, obesity and diabetes have reached epidemic levels worldwide, and they now pose enormous health and socioeconomic challenges. One response to the epidemic has been an outpouring of ideas—including lots of misinformation—about how obesity develops and the best ways to treat it. In this book, my goal is to counter the myths and misinformation while providing the facts and knowledge that people need to control their weight and maintain adequate health. I'll highlight the scope of the problem, discuss fundamental science, dispel myths, and offer practical strategies for treatment and prevention. Better understanding and the will to act on that understanding are the keys to ending the obesity crisis.

Can the Obesity Crisis
Be Reversed?

Struggling with Obesity

OVER THE DECADES that I have been studying and treating obesity, I've met many patients who are struggling to lose weight or control their diabetes and related illnesses. Every patient is different, but here's a composite portrait that draws on some of the difficulties they typically face.

Growing up, Ruth was always one of the bigger girls in her class. She was plump even as a baby, and during her childhood her family fed her a steady diet of processed foods, restaurant meals, red meat, and dairy products. But it was not until she was a teenager that she became self-conscious about her size, mainly because of the bullying she received during gym class.

During her senior year in high school, Ruth made a promise to herself to lose her excess weight before beginning college. She started taking long walks and gradually worked her way up to jogging five miles without a break. On the recommendation of a health information website, Ruth reduced her food intake to 1,200 calories per day. Even though she was constantly hungry, she managed to stick with her diet for months.

When she entered college, Ruth was 20 pounds lighter than she had been the year before, and she was determined to keep the weight off. But maintaining her diet in college was increasingly difficult. Balancing schoolwork and campus life was stressful, especially being away from her family, and the anxiety made her even more fixated on her constant hunger. Eventually, it got to the point that she couldn't concentrate on anything else. One night after everyone had gone to sleep, she raided her dorm's vending machine and ate until she thought she was going to be sick.

Although she told herself it was just a one-time lapse, during the following weeks she had a couple more binging episodes. Then something wonderful and unexpected happened: She started making friends, and the hunger and binging episodes declined as she grew more confident and comfortable in her new circumstances. As her anxiety diminished, she also began worrying less about sticking to her 1,200-calorie diet.

Ruth's weight fluctuated throughout her college years. Going to parties and restaurants with friends was great for her social life, but she gained weight when she stopped paying attention to what she was eating. She and her roommate tried various fad diets, some of which excluded entire food groups. But even though she often managed to lose a few pounds, she always put them back on, plus a few more. Meanwhile, her roommate, who never really needed to diet in the first place, remained thin, even when she seemed to be eating lots of pizza and drinking beer.

When Ruth graduated from college, she went to work as a bookkeeper. She decided to live alone, though she could barely afford a studio apartment. After paying rent, she survived mainly on dollar pizza slices and microwaved meals. She often felt hungry, but her clothes were getting tighter, and she knew she was gaining weight.

To deal with the weight gain, Ruth began jogging again on the weekends. Then, several months into her new routine, she twisted her ankle during a run. The doctor she saw at the local clinic told her that she would have to avoid exercise for at least three months and go to physical therapy.

About that time she met Andrew, and they hit it off right away. Like Ruth, Andrew was overweight, but he didn't worry much about what he ate. Ruth tried to resist the food he kept in his apartment; when they went out for meals, she tried not to eat too much, but a salad wasn't very satisfying when her boyfriend was enjoying a cheeseburger and fries. Andrew had no interest in losing weight and constantly told Ruth that she was beautiful just the way she was. She knew she'd gained weight since they had first met, but she didn't feel nearly as bad about her body as she once did, even when she learned at a follow-up doctor's appointment that her blood pressure was high.

Ruth and Andrew got engaged and married, and soon after they were expecting their first child. Ruth gained a lot of weight during the pregnancy, partly out of anxiety about this big, expensive change in their lives. By the time her daughter was born,

Ruth was 50 pounds heavier than she had ever been. Although some of that weight came off in the following months, she was left with an additional 20 pounds that would not budge, even as she tried to eat as healthfully as she could while nursing her daughter.

As her daughter, and then later a son, got older, Ruth's life was consumed with errands, play dates, and sports matches. Her son was an extremely picky eater, having little taste for anything but junk food despite her best efforts to feed him healthy meals. Eventually, she grew tired of the constant battle and caved in to his demands. Like her, both her children were on the heavier side, despite engaging in regular physical activity, and Ruth worried about them facing the same bullying from their peers as she once did. Many nights after her children were in bed she found herself worrying about their future while snacking on the potato chips and other junk food that everyone in her family loved.

By the time Ruth's children headed off to college, neither of them had lost their excess weight, and she knew how hard it was for them to feel confident in their bodies. She was convinced that she had given them this curse, and she felt guilty for not being able to help them more. But over the years, she hadn't even been able to keep herself from gaining weight. She wished that someone would tell her how much she needed to eat to not gain weight, but every article she read said something different.

With more time for herself after her children were in college, Ruth forced herself to go for a medical checkup for the first time in years. When she met with the doctor, he told her that her weight of 239 pounds put her at a body mass index (BMI) of 41, which fell into the category of "severe obesity." She knew she'd gained a lot of weight, but being called obese was a shock. Furthermore, her blood pressure was high, and a few days later her blood work revealed that her blood sugar was high as well—she was now at risk for developing diabetes.

The doctor prescribed a blood pressure medication and put Ruth on a typical weight-loss regimen: eat less, move more. Ruth was crushed. It was the same advice she had been trying to follow her whole life without success. She mentioned this to the doctor, but he dismissed her concerns, saying she probably had been eating more than she realized. She wanted to lose weight, but after all she had been through she wondered whether it was possible.

"How did I get here?" Ruth asked herself. Was her body weight predetermined, or was it all her fault? And why did she have to go through this when she had many thin friends who could eat whatever they wanted and never gain a pound?

THE BIG PICTURE

Ruth can't see the big picture, but we can. She didn't choose to become obese, nor was her weight gain the result of some personal failing. In fact, the truth is quite the opposite. Ruth has actively struggled with her weight for her entire life, and she has engaged in more healthy activities than many "normal weight" people do. Ruth's weight is a product of both her nature and her nurture. Like many people, Ruth's family has a genetic predisposition toward obesity. She was raised during a time when America's food environment was undergoing massive changes. And she sometimes overate in part to cope with lifelong weight-based stigmatization and shame.

Ruth's story helps illustrate the complex ways in which obesity develops and interacts with various genetic factors and with the forces in our environments that promote weight gain. In chapter 1 of this book, I'll look at these factors to better illustrate the many ways in which nature and nurture contribute to obesity. In chapter 2, I'll consider in more detail the environmental factors that have caused so many people to gain weight over the past few decades.

Although Ruth's battle with weight gain is her own, many people face very similar struggles, failures, and resignation. Why do so many people struggle with their weight and fail? How do commonalities among their stories help to illuminate new potentials for treatment?

RISING NUMBERS

A significant number of people in the United States and around the world find themselves in situations comparable to Ruth's. In the 1960s and '70s, only about one in every seven Americans was obese—that is, they had a body mass index greater than 30 (see "The Body Mass Index: Its Strengths and Weaknesses" on page 8). Today, four of every ten American adults are obese—a total of more than 100 million people—and another three in ten are overweight.[1] About 10 percent of US adults are severely obese, a percentage that has risen tenfold since the 1970s. More Americans now live with severe obesity than with breast cancer, Parkinson's disease, Alzheimer's disease, and HIV combined.[2]

Although obesity affects people from all walks of life, the percentage of people with obesity varies across groups. Socially and economically disadvantaged groups, including some racial and ethnic minorities, have higher rates of obesity than do other groups. These disparities are caused by an interrelated set of social and economic injustices. These groups have higher rates of unemployment, higher levels of food insecurity, and less access to convenient places for physical activity, and they are the object of targeted marketing of unhealthy foods, all of which increase the risk for obesity. They also have less access to health care and face biased treatment when they do receive care, which means they have fewer opportunities to prevent or treat weight gain. Prejudice against people who are obese compounds and reinforces the other disadvantages that members of these groups face.

As my fellow Bloomberg Distinguished Professor Jessica Fanzo has pointed out, many of the same people who struggle with extra weight also regularly go to bed hungry. At first glance, this may seem like an impossible paradox, but on closer examination, it becomes clear that poverty connects these two

The Body Mass Index:
Its Strengths and Weaknesses

The number most often used today to measure body fat is the body mass index (BMI), but it was originally designed for a different purpose. In the early nineteenth century, the Belgian astronomer, mathematician, statistician, and sociologist Adolphe Quetelet originated the idea of dividing a person's height by the square of that person's weight as a way of measuring "the average man."

In 1972, the American physiologist Ancel Keys, best known for his groundbreaking studies on cholesterol and cardiovascular health, proposed that Quetelet's measure be named the "body mass index." The term became widely used when it was observed to correlate with measures of body fat and with the health status of children.

Currently, US government guidelines define a healthy weight as a BMI of 18.5 up to 24.9. People who are overweight have a BMI of 25 to 29.9. A BMI of 30 or above is considered obese, with extreme or severe obesity defined as a BMI above 40.

The body mass index is far from a perfect measure, as it does not accurately measure fat content, reflect the proportions of muscle and fat, or account for gender and racial differences in fat content and distribution. For instance, muscle weighs more than fat; hence, athletes often have the same BMIs as those who are overweight, when in fact they are lean. Furthermore, because of the differences in body composition between men and women, women typically have a significantly higher percentage of body fat than men even when they have the same BMI. In addition, older people tend to have a higher percentage of body fat than do younger people at the same BMI because body composition changes with age. To put it simply, a given BMI may be numerically the same for two individuals, but this number may not represent the same percentage of body fat, the same degree of risk, or even the same degree of overweight or obesity.

Measuring children's BMI is also problematic. In the United States, the Centers for Disease Control and Prevention define a child whose BMI falls between the 85th and the 94th percentile for age and gender as overweight. A child whose BMI is at the 95th percentile or higher for their age and gender is defined as obese. But body fat differs at different ages and between genders. In children and teens, the healthy range for BMI varies by gender.

Any single measure of excess body fat has limitations. As with other metrics used in medicine, such indicators must be combined with other physical and laboratory health information to assess an individual's risk of developing diabetes, heart disease, and other diseases. Nevertheless, the BMI and other measures can be useful tools in managing the health of individuals and populations.

circumstances. People who lack food security struggle to eat a healthy diet, as nutritious foods are often more expensive and less calorically dense than processed and fast foods. Many people who live in low-income areas are also sedentary as a result of their built environments. These areas typically have high concentrations of fast-food restaurants and convenience stores and fewer grocery stores selling fresh, affordable food. Combined, the far-reaching social and environmental consequences of poverty drive higher obesity rates among disadvantaged groups in America.

Without significant changes, the percentages of people who are overweight or obese in the United States will continue to climb. A study in the *New England Journal of Medicine* predicted that more than half of the US population will be obese by 2030, and nearly one in four will be severely obese.[3] The rates are likely to be even higher among women, low-income adults, and non-Hispanic Black adults. According to the study, the prevalence of obesity will approach 60 percent in some states and not dip below 35 percent in any state.

A WORLDWIDE PROBLEM

Once a problem afflicting wealthier countries like the United States, obesity now affects every country in the world. Since 1980, the obesity rate has doubled in 73 countries, has increased in 113 others, and has decreased in none.[4] The largest increases in obesity since 1980 have occurred in low- and middle-income countries, particularly in urban settings in Oceania, Latin America, and North America. If nothing is done to reverse current trends, by 2030 more than two billion adults will be overweight, and more than one billion adults will be obese.[5]

Much of this increase in obesity worldwide can be attributed to globalization. Trade liberalization has provided people access to many types of food, primarily in the form of high-calorie processed foods. It has also allowed multinational food companies and fast-food chains to expand into low-income countries. Globalization has had immense benefits for many people around the world. It has lifted millions of people out of poverty, reduced hunger and infectious disease, and improved quality of life. At the same time, food consumption has shifted from traditional diets to so-called Western diets, characterized by high amounts of processed meat, prepackaged foods, candy and sweets, fried foods, high-fat dairy products, refined grains, potatoes, corn, and high-sugar drinks. Just as in the United States and other wealthy countries, these changes in eating patterns have contributed to a precipitous rise in rates of obesity.

Urbanization has also contributed to the rise in obesity. Currently, more than half of the world's population lives in cities compared with just 10 percent in 1900.[6] Countries that were primarily rural in the past are experiencing this urban transition at astounding rates. In China, more than a billion people will be living in urban centers by 2050—more than double the number of people who live in cities today. Like globalization, urbanization has its pros and cons. Urbanization provides easier access to health care and education, two systems that can help to curb obesity rates. However, city living can also lead to poorer diets, less physical activity, and increased weight. In many countries, urbanization is occurring so quickly that these vital support services are inadequately developed.

THE TOLL ON HEALTH

As obesity rates have increased, so have the rates of health problems related to obesity, as I'll discuss in chapter 3. Being obese increases a person's risk of developing diabetes, hypertension, coronary artery disease, strokes, sleep apnea, gallstones, cirrhosis of the liver, arthritis, low fertility, dementia, and some kinds of cancer. The lifetime risk of premature death for an adult with obesity is more than double that of someone who is not obese. The more obese people are, the more likely they are to die from a heart attack. (The same applies to COVID-19, as I'll discuss in the final chapter of this book.) A Columbia University study from 2013 indicated that obesity accounts for nearly one in every five deaths among Americans between ages 40 and 85, from a number of related causes.[7] Around the world, excess weight plays a role in many millions of deaths every year.

Obesity is costly not only to our health but to our economy as well. Many people are less productive because of excess weight. Many of the people whom I help treat at Johns Hopkins don't work because they're functionally disabled by their obesity—and they're often young people. Treating obesity and obesity-related conditions costs billions of dollars a year, and these costs continue to grow as more people become obese.[8] In 2015, obesity-related medical costs accounted for 7.91 percent of all US national medical expenditures, a 29 percent increase from 2001.[9] If we continue along our current path, experts estimate these costs will total between $48 billion and $66 billion a year in the United States by 2030.[10] These direct costs include outpatient and inpatient health services (including surgery), laboratory and radiological tests, and drug therapies related to treating obesity and its associated comorbidities.

Again, the burden falls hardest on some population groups. Not only do certain racial and ethnic groups have higher rates of obesity, but they also face worse prospects in receiving adequate care. Both non-Hispanic Blacks and Hispanics face discrimination in accessing and receiving adequate health care services. Combined with the stigmatization that people who are obese encounter in health care settings, these groups are at a significant disadvantage in getting proper treatment for obesity and its related health conditions.

IS THE RISE IN OBESITY AN EPIDEMIC?

After two decades of rising trends in obesity, the World Health Organization (WHO) convened an expert consultation in 1997 that determined that the world is in the midst of an obesity "epidemic." But is the rise in obesity rates, which has continued since then, truly an epidemic?

The term *epidemic* describes the occurrence of a disease that is spreading rapidly. In turn, a disease is a medical condition that has a cause, a diagnosis, a course of progression, and usually a treatment. By this definition, obesity is a disease, in that it is a medical condition that can harm health. And because obesity has been spreading so rapidly, I believe the use of the term *epidemic* is appropriate, despite the term's severity.

In fact, the severity that the word implies is precisely the point. Obesity is a serious problem, and we must take it seriously to prevent needless morbidity and mortality. After all, most people now live in countries where being overweight or obese kills more individuals than do starvation and undernutrition.

At the same time, the word *epidemic* may erroneously imply that obesity has straightforward causes and therefore simple cures. To the contrary, obesity is a very complex condition, with new advances continually being made to unravel its origins and improve treatment options. As I'll discuss throughout this book, obesity is a chronic illness that can be managed but not "cured" in the strict sense of the word. In that respect, long-term interventions are essential to help people who are obese lose weight in an effective, sustainable, and conscientious way, as I'll discuss in chapter 4.

A CRITICAL JUNCTURE

Many people and institutions still consider obesity a problem of personal behaviors that could be reversed by simply deciding to eat less and exercise more. But this is the wrong way of looking at it. As with other chronic diseases, obesity has complicated origins and complicated solutions. People cannot control many of the factors that make them gain weight. As I'll discuss in chapter 5, they need help and support from their families and friends, communities, governments, and the broader society in order to achieve success.

As a result of new discoveries in basic, clinical, and population sciences, this is a particularly opportune time to take on the challenges of obesity and associated diseases. Researchers have made major advances in understanding and treating obesity, partly due to extensive animal studies, research in human populations, and fundamental biological research. Public awareness and policymakers' interest in doing something about obesity have also increased. Several groups, including the American Medical Association, the American Diabetes Association, and the American Heart Association have recognized obesity as a disease, further reinforcing the need for effective, long-term, and safe treatment options.

Reversing the obesity epidemic will require a commitment from all involved. Researchers must continue to study the ways in which obesity develops and affects the body. Doctors must provide more comprehensive, more engaged, and less judgmental treatment for patients with obesity. People who are obese must commit to getting treatment and making lifestyle changes. Communities must make efforts to have affordable, healthy foods available for purchase. Governments must create policies that promote healthy weight. Every sector and every person will be important in treating and preventing obesity. We must all act now to address the causes, consequences, prevention, and treatment of obesity.

CHAPTER 1

How Do People Gain Excess Weight?

THE OBESITY PROBLEM IS COMPLEX and yet logical. When people consume more food energy than they burn, the net result is excess energy, which is stored mainly as body fat. If people create a sustained energy deficit by eating less and/or expending more energy, they will lose weight.

But losing weight and keeping it off is almost never simple; nor is it simply a matter of personal willpower. For example, the amount of energy that a person uses each day depends on many factors, including genetics, age, gender, muscle-to-fat ratio, physical activity, underlying medical conditions, the nutrient composition of food, and gut microbes. With so many factors at play, how to balance food intake against our body's energy requirements is far from obvious.

Treating obesity also involves much more than simply reducing caloric intake. It depends on many aspects of a person's lifestyle, a wide variety of influences in that person's environment, health status, and other factors. Effective treatment therefore requires an understanding of the complex drivers that contribute to excess weight and attention to the unique factors characteristic of each individual.

FROM FOOD TO FAT

People need a continuous source of energy to stay alive, but eating occurs intermittently over the course of the day. Since energy cannot be created or destroyed, animals like us need mechanisms to match this episodic supply of food with the constant requirement for the energy that fuels our bodies.

A major mechanism that allows us to get from one meal to the next is the storage of the sugar glucose in a complex form as glycogen ("animal starch"), mainly in the liver and muscles. A useful analogy for this system is a bank account. Money is periodically deposited into the account (similar to food intake), where it's stored temporarily and depleted by continuous spending. The presence of the bank account acts as a buffer between intermittent earning of income and a constant need to spend money.

However, animals also need long-term storage mechanisms to tide them over when they can't get enough food to meet their bodies' demands. This mechanism is provided by fat stored mainly in fat tissues, which are also known as adipose tissues. Extending the analogy, body fat is like a savings account. During periods when food is abundantly available, animals can deposit energy into body fat so that it is available for periods when demand exceeds supply.

When we eat, the process of converting food to fat storage

begins. All the foods we eat are composed of varying proportions of three macronutrients—carbohydrates, protein, and fat. These macronutrients supply varying levels of energy to the body, with each unit of energy commonly known as a calorie. Carbohydrates and proteins both provide about 4 calories per gram; fats provide about 9 calories per gram. Thus, it makes sense that a hamburger, which is high in fat, has more calories than a grapefruit, which is high in carbohydrates and water.

However, before our body can use these three macronutrients for energy, they must be broken down into smaller molecules. This is the process that occurs during digestion. Enzymes in the gut facilitate this process, transforming carbohydrates into glucose, proteins into their constituent amino acids, and fats into fatty acids and glycerol. Most of these nutrients travel through the bloodstream to the liver, which further processes them while screening out harmful substances. The liver then directs these nutrients to the rest of the body for use or storage.

If our bodies have more fatty acids than they currently need, the remainder are sent to adipose tissue to be stored. Adipose tissue can store a huge number of calories. Most people can survive for three to four months without eating so long as they consume fluids because adipose tissues store enough calories to sustain them. To put it in perspective, the liver stores roughly 450 calories of fat at any time, while muscle stores around 3,000 calories of fat. The 35 pounds of fat in a 180-pound person with 20 percent body fat are the equivalent of more than 120,000 calories. There is nothing wrong with fat—it is the critical tissue that allows us to maintain our energy. It's excess fat that's worrisome.

In addition to providing us with the nutrients needed for optimal health, our diets must meet our energy requirements. A state of healthy energy balance is attained when dietary energy intake is equal to energy expenditure—a condition known as homeostasis. A person will remain at a steady weight when the energy balance is maintained over a long period.

When you lose weight, it's because your fat cells, or adipocytes, are providing more energy to the body than they are receiving. As a result, the adipocytes become smaller and you become lighter. However, you may not actually lose adipocytes during this process. Instead, your adipocytes just shrink. Conversely, when you gain weight, your adipocytes accumulate fat and become larger. Essentially, the body is constantly making and using fat. Whether you gain, lose, or maintain body fat and weight depends on the rate of making to using fat.

THE ROLE OF METABOLISM

Many people talk about metabolism as if it were a muscle or an organ in our body. They might say that they have a "good" metabolism that burns energy quickly or a "bad" metabolism that makes it more difficult to lose weight.

In reality, metabolism refers to the process I just described, of converting nutrients into energy that the body uses. Thousands of biochemical reactions are involved in metabolic processes, and these reactions are affected by both our genetics and our environments. Just as obesity is a product of both nature and nurture, so is metabolism.

Your metabolism is always working. Even when you sleep, your body is still burning energy for functions like breathing, circulating blood, and repairing cells. The energy that your body uses for these basic functions when you are not moving is called your basal metabolic rate. This basal metabolic rate accounts for the majority of the total calories that you burn each day (between 65 and 80 percent for adults). Physical activity accounts for 10 to 30 percent of your daily energy expenditure. Diet-induced thermogenesis, which is the heat generated to digest the food that you eat, accounts for roughly 10 percent of daily energy expenditure.

A "slow metabolism" is frequently blamed for weight gain, just as people who are naturally slim often claim to have fast metabolisms. But can we really blame obesity on a slow metabolism? Laboratory and clinical studies indicate that a slow metabolism is not the main culprit for weight gain in most people. Furthermore, efforts to speed up your metabolism are not an effective way to lose weight in most people. Although certain foods like coffee, chili, and other spices may speed up the metabolic rate, the change is so small and short-lived that it would not be enough to produce sustained weight loss.

Even though a slow metabolism is not a major cause of obesity in most people, metabolic rates do differ from person to person depending on a variety of factors. First, as mentioned above, metabolism depends largely on a person's basal metabolic rate. In turn, this basal metabolic rate is influenced by age, sex, body size, and body composition. If you weigh more or have more muscle mass, you will burn more calories, even at rest. As a result, people who weigh more actually have a higher basal metabolic rate rather than a lower one.

Sex is also an important determinant of metabolic rate. Men tend to have less body fat and more muscle mass than do women of the same age and height, and they therefore tend to burn more calories. Also, as people age, they lose muscle mass and accrue fat. Fat burns fewer calories at rest than muscles, so older people tend to burn fewer calories than they did when they were younger.

The take-home message is that our metabolic rates are different, depending on who we are as individuals. Our metabolic rates are always changing depending on the basic energy needs of the body, physical activities, and health status. Whether there is excess energy for storage as fat is determined by the balance of how much food a person eats and how much energy is expended. This is why weight gain varies so much from one person to another.

HORMONES AND OUR DIETS

Hormones control feeding and metabolism, and they play major roles in the processing of energy from food. For example, the hormone insulin, which is produced by the pancreas, acts as a signal to our bodies to store energy in the forms of glycogen, protein, and fat. When the pancreas senses an increase in blood sugar levels caused by the consumption of food, it releases insulin, which drives glucose to enter our cells for use as a fuel.

Sometimes the insulin-producing cells are destroyed by an autoimmune process. In this case, a lack of insulin leads to very high blood glucose levels, frequent urination, and excessive thirst. This disease, known as type 1 diabetes, can be deadly if not treated promptly with insulin injections.

In another form of diabetes, known as type 2 diabetes, the body does not produce enough insulin to move glucose into cells, or cells become resistant to the influence of insulin. As a result, the amount of sugar in the bloodstream continues to rise, resulting in hyperglycemia (high blood sugar) and preventing the body from using sugar for energy. Unlike type 1 diabetes, people with type 2 diabetes can live with the disease for many years with few or no symptoms. In patients like Ruth, weight gain is associated with insulin resistance and increasing blood glucose levels (pre-diabetes). Unless she loses weight, her pre-diabetes will progress to type 2 diabetes, causing major damage to the heart, blood vessels, eyes, kidneys, and nerves if left untreated.

While important, insulin is far from the only hormone involved in energy and weight regulation. As I noted in the preface, since the discovery of leptin in 1994, researchers have known that adipose tissue actively produces various hormones that play a role in the body's digestion and storage of food energy. Adipose tissue thus has a direct link both to the body's metabolic processes and to obesity.

One thing we've discovered is that the release of hormones from adipose tissue and other organs can have various metabolic effects. Leptin is produced in proportion to body fat. In humans and mice lacking leptin, leptin deficiency drives appetite and weight gain, and leptin treatment reduces appetite and prevents weight gain. Low leptin levels activate areas in the brain that control satiety, food reward, and metabolism. In most people with obesity, such as Ruth, their adipose tissues produce excessive amounts of leptin, yet the rise in leptin does not reduce their appetite or prevent weight gain. Research in animals and humans indicates that obesity is commonly associated with leptin resistance. Whether leptin resistance directly drives weight increase in obesity is less clear, but studies have suggested that the fall in leptin during weight loss in people with obesity is a significant stimulator of eating and weight regain. This may explain why patients like Ruth have great difficulty maintaining weight loss.

Another important hormone is called ghrelin, which is secreted by the stomach and increases appetite. Research suggests that ghrelin is a meal initiator. Throughout the day, ghrelin levels fluctuate, sharply rising before scheduled mealtimes and then falling after eating. When ghrelin rises, the brain senses hunger and stimulates feeding. Furthermore, ghrelin activates pathways that increase the motivation to eat and the rewarding sensations experienced from eating. In contrast to leptin levels, which rise in people with obesity, ghrelin levels vary among people with obesity. However, some studies have suggested that the suppression of ghrelin after eating a meal is blunted in people with obesity; that may be one reason why these individuals might still feel hungry even after eating.

The location of fat in the body also affects our hormones. People have a tendency to store fat in different locations. Some people accumulate fat around their liver and other abdominal organs, which is known as visceral fat (also called central obesity). Others tend to store fat just below the skin, known as subcutaneous fat. People who carry large amounts of visceral fat often have excess weight around the midsection, while excess subcutaneous fat tends to concentrate around the hips, thighs, and buttocks. Although visceral fat accounts for a small proportion of the body fat in a person with a normal BMI, a person with obesity can have a much higher level of visceral fat, and this is the type of fat that is most worrisome. Visceral fat is associated with insulin resistance, diabetes, and an increased risk of cardiovascular disease, dementia, breast cancer, and colorectal cancer. Excessive visceral fat predisposes an individual to developing "metabolic syndrome," which is characterized by elevated glucose and triglyceride levels in the blood, high blood pressure, and reduced levels of high-density lipoprotein (so-called good cholesterol) in the blood. The risk of metabolic syndrome is increased in older men and post-menopausal women. Studies have shown that excess subcutaneous fat—for example, in young women—protects against diabetes and heart disease.

Eating is also influenced by the sight, smell, and taste of food, thinking about food, sleeping or waking, stress, and environmental and social factors. For example, during a buffet meal, people may consume large amounts of food and drinks not because they are hungry but because they are enjoying the company of friends. Even after you feel full, your desire to eat more can be driven by how delicious a meal is, how the meal is presented, or whether the situation is fun, such as a Superbowl party. On the other hand, you may not want to eat even when you're hungry—for instance, when you're feeling sick, anxious, or sad or when the food smells bad or tastes terrible. While "hunger eating" is controlled by hormonal and gut signals to the hypothalamus, hedonic (pleasure) eating is controlled by areas of the brain connected to mood and behavior. In modern societies where food is plentiful, affordable, and palatable, hedonic eating is often underappreciated as a driver of obesity and associated diseases.

GENETICS OF OBESITY

We know that genetics has a role in the development of obesity, since genes influence almost every aspect of human life. In rare cases, malfunctions in just one or a handful of genes cause obesity. But in the vast majority of cases, hundreds or thousands of genes are involved, mostly having small effects. Though much remains unknown, great progress has been made in understanding these genetic influences on obesity.

When I see a young patient who is complaining of severe hunger, uncontrolled eating, and rapid weight gain, I have to consider whether a mutation in a single gene might be responsible—so-called monogenic obesity. Such mutations have been discovered in genes that play essential roles in regulating food intake and energy homeostasis, such as the genes that code for leptin and for the leptin receptor. Obesity is also a hallmark of some chromosomal abnormalities that are accompanied by intellectual impairment, reproductive anomalies, congenital organ defects, limb or facial dysmorphism, and endocrine dysfunction. In cases where monogenic obesity occurs, the mother and father are often related to each other in some way; therefore, assessment of the family tree is essential in such a diagnosis.

The discovery of leptin was an important milestone in the understanding of monogenic obesity. Leptin, named after the Greek word *leptos*, meaning to be thin, was originally thought to act in the brain to inhibit food intake and decrease body weight. This hypothesis was driven by the discovery that mice lacking a functional gene for leptin were unable to suppress their feeding and gained excessive weight. Furthermore, follow-up studies showed that when leptin-deficient mice were treated with the hormone they lacked, their obesity was cured.[1]

As do mice, human patients lacking a functional leptin gene

develop a voracious appetite, morbid obesity, and hormonal abnormalities, all of which are effectively cured by leptin treatment. This finding was the first definitive proof that hormones made by adipose tissue are critical to our body's regulation of weight.

However, unlike congenital leptin deficiency, most people with obesity are not leptin deficient. On the contrary, obesity is commonly associated with *higher* levels of leptin than in thinner people, making leptin treatment an unsuitable option. In important research studies conducted on mice during my fellowship training under Jeffrey Flier, we discovered that leptin's primary function is to signal starvation to the brain. When rodents lose weight from food deprivation, leptin levels fall rapidly and trigger adaptive responses. Brain activity increases in the hypothalamus and other areas involved in the regulatory, emotional, cognitive, and sensory control of food intake. This leads to greater levels of eating and reduced energy expenditures, which leads to restoration of energy stores and weight. This is one reason why it's very common for people to regain weight they have lost. When people are on severely restricted diets, their leptin levels fall rapidly and they are very hungry. Thus, failure to maintain weight loss is not purely the result of a lack of willpower. Instead, it's a product of the body's coordinated biological response to weight loss that causes changes in appetite and metabolism.

Perhaps the mechanisms mediated through reduced leptin levels evolved as a protection against the threat of starvation by limiting energy use and enhancing fat storage. However, in our modern environment, where food is plentiful and opportunities for exercise are sparse, this metabolic efficiency may predispose us toward obesity (see "Why Did Evolution Predispose Us to Obesity?" on page 30).

THE INFLUENCE OF MANY GENES

Although research into monogenic obesity has greatly improved our understanding of the genes that relate to various aspects of weight regulation, these studies can only tell us so much. For most people, obesity is a product of hundreds or even thousands of genetic variants working together to control eating and metabolism; so-called common obesity is related to polygenic factors. The effects of any one gene may be very small, but many people inherit collections of genetic variants that predispose them toward excess weight if they are in environments that promote weight gain.

Many of the genetic variants identified in these studies are expressed in the brain, and some have been shown to regulate feeding and body weight in animal models. The effect of many common genetic variants can be combined into a "polygenic risk score" that predicts a person's risk of becoming obese. However, all the common genetic variants associated with obesity have modest effects.

Studies of twins also offer some insight into the contribution

Why Did Evolution Predispose Us to Obesity?

The origins of obesity are much better understood than they were a few decades ago, but much remains unknown. One big question is why would evolution favor a condition that has so many negative consequences?

Three primary explanations have been offered.[1] The first hypothesis is that obesity might have increased the odds of survival in the past by allowing our ancestors to endure periods of famine. For example, people with so-called thrifty genes may have been better at gaining weight between periods of famine, but limited food supplies kept them from gaining enough weight to experience the detrimental health outcomes associated with obesity. Then, during the twentieth century, as a result of improvements in agriculture, food became more available throughout Europe and North America and gradually spread across the rest of the world. Although famines remain a feature of some low-income nations, they are rarer than before. As a result, people with these "thrifty genes" deposit fat in anticipation of a famine that never arrives, thus predisposing them toward obesity.

However, if thrifty genes provide a strong selective advantage to surviving famine, and if famines have occurred regularly throughout human history, then by now all of us would have inherited these "thrifty genes," and all of us would be obese. But even among the most obese societies in the world, like the US, roughly 20 percent of the population remains lean, calling into question the thrifty gene hypothesis.

The second evolutionary hypothesis posits that obesity may have been nonexistent in our evolutionary past, except perhaps in some rare genetic cases. Its prevalence today is instead a by-product of positive selection on some other advantageous trait. For example, maybe evolution favored the development in cold climates of a kind of fat tissue known as brown adipose tissue (BAT), which burns off calories in the process of producing body heat.

However, such explanations also have problems. In the case of BAT, humans have many other ways of burning calories. And the genes currently known to be associated with obesity do not appear to be linked with the function of BAT.

The third evolutionary hypothesis proposes a neutral explanation for the obesity epidemic. According to this view, obesity has not been subject to strong selection in the past. Instead, the genes that predispose us to obesity have been changing randomly over evolutionary time, and these random changes have made some individuals prone to obesity and others resistant to it.

Of these three hypotheses, the neutral explanation may be the most valid. However, it is probably best not to place undue emphasis on any one of these hypotheses, since the current obesity epidemic cannot be blamed on evolutionary processes acting in isolation. These ideas are interesting, but they tend to oversimplify the complexities underlying obesity and fail to account for the many other features of modern society that interact with body weight and energy balance.

NOTE

1. John R. Speakman. 2013. Evolutionary perspectives on the obesity epidemic: adaptive, maladaptive, and neutral viewpoints. *Annual Review of Nutrition* 33: 289–317.

of heredity to obesity. Identical twins tend to have similar body weights, whereas fraternal twins tend to have weights similar to those of siblings who are not twins.[2] This indicates that the genes people inherit from their parents undoubtedly play some role in determining their weight.

Genetic researchers used to think that careful study of the genes that cause monogenic obesity would explain many of the mechanisms behind polygenic obesity. However, this has turned out not to be the case. Common obesity involves far more genes and environmental interactions than previously thought. Though monogenic forms of obesity offer interesting insights into the development of obesity, they are far from the whole story.

Furthermore, genetic factors are unlikely to explain the recent surge in obesity rates. The frequency of different genes in the human gene pool has remained relatively stable for generations. A person's genes may increase the risk of obesity, but the environment determines whether that risk will be realized. Someone begins working the night shift, starts sleeping poorly and eating at odd times, and steadily gains weight. People go to work in places where they sit all day, eat calorie-rich food from a cafeteria, and can't even walk around the block during breaks. A fetus grows in the uterus of a mother who has diabetes or obesity and is exposed to biochemical influences that result in gaining extra weight after birth. Meanwhile, other people who have genetic variants that predispose to obesity do not become overweight because they eat well and stay active.

OBESITY ASSOCIATED
WITH MEDICAL CONDITIONS

Unlike "common" obesity, rapid weight gain may accompany various medical conditions. Obesity can result from hormonal disorders, such as in patients with thyroid hormone deficiency, excess cortisol, or excess estrogen. When you make too little thyroid hormone, your metabolic rate is reduced and you gain weight. High doses of glucocorticoids used to treat chronic lung diseases, rheumatological disorders, or cancer can cause people to gain weight, mainly in the center of the body. These people also have decreased muscle strength and skin that bruises easily, factors that tend to discourage physical activity and result in further weight gain. Similarly, Cushing syndrome, which arises from excess cortisol production by the adrenal gland, causes central obesity, muscle weakness in the thighs and shoulders, bruising, and diabetes. Insulin, which is commonly used to treat patients who are obese and have type 2 diabetes, is also a growth factor, so these patients tend to gain extra weight.

Estrogen given as an oral contraceptive can cause weight gain. Similarly, most patients with polycystic ovarian syndrome are obese. In rare cases, people who sustain head injuries can damage their hypothalamus, which can lead to reduced levels of sex hormones, thyroid hormone, or growth hormone, low energy expenditure, and weight gain. Injury to the hypothalamus, for example, from a tumor or fracture of the base of the

MEDICATIONS ASSOCIATED WITH OBESITY

DISEASE	MEDICATION CLASS	MEDICATION NAMES	ALTERNATIVE MEDICATIONS
Diabetes	Hypertension	Human insulin Insulin analogs	There is no alternative for insulin therapy in patients with type 1 diabetes. For patients with type 2 diabetes, metformin and DPP4 inhibitors do not cause weight gain; GLP-1 receptor agonists and SGLT-2 inhibitors may reduce weight.
	Sulfonylureas	Chlorpropamide Glimepiride Glipizide Glyburide Tolbutamide	
	Thiazolidinediones	Pioglitazone	
Depression	Tricyclic antidepressants	Amytriptyline Doxepine Imipramine Mirtazapine Nortriptyline Trimipramine	Bupropion Nefazodone
	Lithium	Lithium	
	Selective Serotonin Reuptake Inhibitors (SSRIs)	Fluvoxamine Paroxetine Sertraline	SSRIs can cause initial weight loss, followed by weight gain in a few patients.
Psychosis; schizophrenia	Antipsychotics	Chlorpromazine Clozapine Fluphenazine Haloperidol Loxapine Olanzapine Quetiapine Risperidone	Ziprasidone
Epilepsy; seizures	Antiseizure medications; anticonvulsants	Carbamazepine Gabapentin Valproic Acid	Lamotrigine Topiramate Zonisamide
Inflammatory diseases; cancer	Glucocorticoids	Dexamethasone Prednisone	
Asthma; chronic obstructive pulmonary disease	Glucocorticoids (inhaled)	Budesonide Ciclesonide Fluticasone	
Contraception	Sex steroids	Estrogen Progestagen	
Allergy	Antihistamines	Diphenhydramine	
Hypertension	Beta blockers	Atenolol Metoprolol Propranolol	Angiotensin-converting enzyme (ACE) inhibitors; angiotensin II receptor blockers (ARB); calcium channel blockers

skull, results in voracious appetite, overeating, and weight gain. Finally, just as rarely, some people have tumors that secrete excessive amounts of insulin. The high insulin produced by insulin-secreting tumors (insulinomas) drastically lowers blood glucose, stimulates food intake, and causes rapid weight gain. Fortunately, the majority of insulinomas are not cancerous, and removing the tumors typically resolves their effects on the body and enables complete recovery.

Apart from hormonal therapies, some commonly prescribed medications are associated with weight gain (see the table). Drug side effects may include increased appetite, reduced energy expenditure, or disrupted glucose and fat metabolism. Some medications may cause fatigue or sleepiness, making it difficult for people to exercise. Other medications can promote water retention, which increases body weight but not fat. These side effects vary from person to person, and because the medications are often taken for chronic diseases, the weight gain may persist for several years.

Patients need to ask their doctors whether a newly prescribed medication is known to cause weight gain and whether there are alternative medications that do not increase weight. Weight gain typically occurs within six months after starting a new medication; therefore, it is important to monitor your weight and alert your doctor. Ultimately, the risk for weight gain needs to be balanced against the effectiveness of the medication.

CHAPTER 2

Why Are People Getting Heavier?

NOW THAT WE KNOW MORE about how obesity develops, let's return to Ruth's story from the introduction. She likely has a genetic propensity to gain weight. She was plump as a child and has struggled with weight issues her whole life, and her children have encountered similar problems. She has lost weight in the past through strenuous dieting, but it tends to come back when she is less vigilant about what she eats.

Still, environmental factors have obviously contributed to Ruth's struggles with obesity. When she was a child, her parents fed her processed and energy-dense foods that caused her to gain weight. Most children who are obese will be obese as adults. In college, Ruth experimented with various fad diets, but she rarely was able to stick with them for long. Meanwhile, she had ready access to highly processed and unhealthy food, whereas healthy foods were less affordable.

Ruth never developed a long-term relationship with a health care professional who could help her manage her diet and physical activity, even when she was diagnosed with high blood pressure and pre-diabetes. She went to doctors when she had an injury and in the course of having children. But the care she got for her weight problem was always reactive—she never received adequate medical and social help.

We'll return to Ruth in chapter 4 and examine some of the health care approaches that could help her remain healthy. The important point for now is that, under different circumstances, Ruth might have had far fewer problems with her weight.

PROCESSED FOOD ENVIRONMENTS

Why have people gotten so much heavier over the past few decades? As I noted in the previous chapter, changes in genetics are not the predominant reason for the obesity epidemic. It has to be something about our environments.

The most obvious change in our environments has to do with the foods we eat. In wealthy and less wealthy countries alike, relatively inexpensive and calorie-dense foods have become almost universally available. They can be bought in supermarkets, convenience stores, bodegas, office buildings, and gas stations. Processed and packaged to have very long shelf lives, junk foods tempt consumers from shelves, vending machines, and home pantries. Our food environments, including the places that advertise and provide access to food, have become increasingly "obesogenic"—they contribute to the development of obesity.

This transformation to obesogenic environments began long

before the explosion of fast-food chains and processed foods. The first domino fell with the agricultural intensification that began in the 1900s. In the first half of the twentieth century, synthetic fertilizers, chemical pesticides, tractors, mechanical harvesters, planters, transplanters, and other tools vastly increased farming efficiencies and crop yields. These innovations, coupled with a growing population and a rising demand for cheap food, caused a huge shift toward maximizing output within the agriculture industry. In the second half of the twentieth century, farms increasingly shifted away from a diverse array of crops to a few high-yielding crops, such as corn and soybeans, grown in massive industrialized operations.

The amount and variety of processed foods also increased rapidly throughout the twentieth century. Processed foods that are altered between the farm and where we eat them were intended to alleviate food shortages and improve the overall nutrition of populations. However, they quickly gained immense popularity for their taste, convenience, and cost, and the industry expanded in many directions beyond its original functions. So-called new and "improved" food products are constantly being released; many of them are promoted by flashy advertising campaigns and offered at increasingly affordable prices. Processed foods currently account for 57 percent of a typical diet in the United States, and that figure continues to rise.[1]

Processed foods are not necessarily bad—if prepared and consumed in healthy ways, they can be useful components of a healthy diet. Such foods include plain yogurt, nut butters, canned beans, veggie burgers, hummus, olive oil, and tofu. However, the ways in which most processed foods are produced, marketed, and distributed inevitably pose risks. First, processed foods tend to have a lot of added sugar and salt with little nutritional value. Also, many processed foods make use of the surplus crops in our food supply, such as corn, wheat, and soy, which are then combined with salt, sugar, fats, and chemical preservatives to enhance their flavor and shelf life. Many consumers don't read the long, tiny, and incomprehensible lists of ingredients on the back of processed foods, which often contain unrecognizable additives such as guar gum, sodium nitrite, carrageenan, and sodium benzoate. Even when they do read these labels, consumers often underestimate the calories, sugar, salt, and portion sizes. Processed foods tend to have very small serving sizes with high energy content—ten potato chips for 170 calories—for instance. But few people actually eat just ten chips at a time. Many people would laugh at how meager ten chips look in a bowl. Instead, people typically consume multiple servings of these high-calorie foods in a single sitting, especially since single packages of processed foods usually contain multiple servings.

FEELING FULL

This leads to the second problem with processed foods. They tend to be less satiating than their whole food counterparts.

Your stomach recognizes fullness based on volume, not caloric density. If you eat a bowl of green vegetables, 20 minutes later your stomach will feel fuller than if you ate a bowl of chips. True, the digestion of these foods occurs in different ways, but it is mainly the bulk of a meal consumed that signals the feeling of fullness. The potato chips are digested quickly, as they provide easy-to-break-down energy, causing a spike in your blood sugar. The green vegetables, on the other hand, are full of fiber, vitamins, and minerals, take longer to digest, and provide your body with more sustained energy as well as valuable nutrients.

A recent study of processed foods and calorie consumption reaffirmed this point.[2] Twenty adults between the ages of 18 and 45 were recruited for the study and moved into the clinical center at the National Institutes of Health for four weeks. There they were divided into two groups. One group ate meals consisting of primarily "ultraprocessed" foods, including ones that many people consider healthy, such as flavored yogurts and processed foods advertised as healthy on their labels. The other group ate mostly unprocessed or minimally processed foods, including oatmeal, roast beef, fresh scrambled eggs, and barley. Each group was offered meals with an equivalent number of calories and proportions of carbohydrates, fat, and sugar. Participants were instructed to eat as much as they wanted, and after two weeks the groups switched diets.

Participants on the ultraprocessed diet consumed an average of 500 more calories a day than did participants on the unprocessed diet, and they gained two pounds over the course of two weeks. On the ultraprocessed diet, participants were found to have increased levels of appetite-stimulating hormones.

A decade ago, I reviewed the book *The End of Overeating* by David A. Kessler, a former commissioner of the Food and Drug Administration who implemented stricter food labeling. In his book, Kessler argues that modern foods, particularly American foods, are designed not to satisfy but rather to stimulate the reward pathways in the brain, much like drugs do, conditioning us to crave more food. In particular, Kessler identified sugar, fat, and salt as the leading culprits of modern food, responsible for heightening our appetites and causing us to gain weight. While I don't agree that the ingredients in modern foods are the only factor involved in the current obesity crisis, they certainly play a major role. My main takeaway from Kessler's book was that the food industry has taken full advantage of our concept of modernity and has increasingly distanced us from the origins of the foods that we eat.

All these changes in food environments serve the food industry's bottom line. The more people eat, the more money the industry makes. Our environments have produced massive profits for these businesses without taking human health into consideration.

SUGAR-SWEETENED BEVERAGES

One type of processed food that has received particular scrutiny for its relation to weight gain is sugar-sweetened beverages.

Research has shown that increases in consumption of these beverages across most age groups in the United States appear to run in parallel to the steep rise in obesity rates.[3] Over the past few decades, US children and adolescents have doubled their daily intake of sugar-sweetened beverages, with similar increases among American adults. This increase in consumption has been closely linked to weight gain over time for both children and adults.

Some experts believe that these products have a special causal relationship with weight gain. The consumption of sugar-sweetened beverages does little to blunt our hunger, potentially causing us to consume more calories than we would otherwise. One reason may be that these beverages cause large insulin spikes within the body, increasing subsequent hunger. Furthermore, the liver metabolizes fructose (from the high-fructose corn syrup in sugar-sweetened beverages) differently than it does glucose (the type of sugar found in whole-grain products), which may result in fat deposition in the liver, insulin resistance, and susceptibility to diabetes.

The evidence linking sugar-sweetened beverages with obesity has resulted in some policy changes, such as higher taxes on these beverages and efforts to eliminate them from schools. Nonetheless, the consumption of sugar-sweetened beverages remains high. In 2012, a quarter of US adults reported consuming at least one such beverage daily.[4] With such a clear correlation between the timing of increased consumption of sugar-sweetened beverages in the United States and the sharp rise of obesity rates, they clearly should be avoided.

FAST FOODS AND FOOD ADVERTISING

Fast-food chains' highly processed foods are ubiquitous across America and, increasingly, around the rest of the world. These restaurants offer hot, tasty, convenient, and cheap meals within minutes. Not surprisingly, research has found that an increase in the consumption of fast food is linked with poorer diet quality and higher energy intake at the individual level. For instance, the CARDIA study, which followed 3,000 young adults for 13 years, found that people who had higher fast-food intake levels at the beginning of the study weighed an average of 13 pounds more than people who had the lowest fast-food intake levels.[5]

What causes this relationship? Like other highly processed foods, fast foods tend to have minimal nutritional value while being high in fat, sugar, and salt. For instance, the typical Big Mac Meal—which comprises a Big Mac burger, a medium order of fries, and a medium soft drink—clocks in at 1,100 calories with 44 grams of fat, 149 grams of carbs, 1,225 milligrams of sodium, and 29 grams of protein. If you order the larger size of fries and a large soft drink, it rises to 1,350 calories, with the extra 250 calories coming from sugar and carbs. For most people, even the regular combo meal contains more than half of the calories that they should eat each day to maintain their weight.

Sugar-sweetened beverages, fast food, and processed foods in general have a particularly detrimental effect on people with low socioeconomic status and from disadvantaged backgrounds. Research has consistently shown that people in poorer communities are surrounded by fast-food restaurants, consume more junk food, and have higher obesity rates.[6] People in these communities often have limited access to the nutritious food options necessary for sustaining a healthy lifestyle. Instead, they live in what are known as "food deserts" or "food swamps" in which it is difficult to buy affordable or good-quality fresh food. More than 2 million US households live in food deserts, without access to cars and farther than a mile from a supermarket. Numerous studies have linked living in food deserts to lower-quality diets and increased risk of obesity.[7] Similarly, food swamps are areas in which fast-food restaurants, junk food outlets, convenience stores, and liquor stores greatly outnumber healthy food options. Both of these environments stand in contrast to "food oases," areas that provide greater access to supermarkets, farmers markets, and shops that stock fresh foods. But these environments tend to exist predominantly in wealthy neighborhoods, once again leaving poor people at greater risk of developing obesity.

Another major presence in many food environments is food advertising. In 2017, food, beverage, and restaurant companies spent nearly $14 billion on advertising in the United States.[8] Food advertising comes in many forms, from highway billboards advertising fast-food restaurants to signs on the sides of skyscrapers depicting six-story-tall celebrities clutching the latest energy drinks. Products are advertised through television commercials and junk mail, but also through sneakier avenues such as product placements, targeted advertisements on social media, "news" stories that are really just promotional ploys, and sponsorships at sports events.

Research has shown that advertisements have the biggest impact on children, who don't have the reasoning abilities to understand the ways in which food advertisements influence viewers.[9] Since children's and adolescents' brains are still developing, they are less able to resist immediate pleasure, like a sweet snack, in favor of a more abstract future benefit like health. Studies have even shown that most children under the age of 6can't distinguish between programming and advertising. This is especially alarming considering that food and beverage companies spend billions of dollars each year to aggressively market foods that are high in sugars, fats, and salts to youth, while there is almost no marketing of fruits, vegetables, and whole grains. Research has also found strong associations between increases in advertising for non-nutritious foods and the rising rates of childhood obesity.

Parents also fall victim to misleading advertisements directed toward children. One study determined that nearly all parents provide sugary drinks to their children, and many believe that some sugary drinks are healthy options for children, especially flavored waters, fruit drinks, and sports drinks.[10] Moreover, many parents rely upon on package claims to determine their purchase decisions. For instance, researchers have found that most parents believe that cereals with nutrition-related claims are more nutritious and healthier for their children, increasing their willingness to buy these cereals despite their questionable nutritional quality.[11] The bottom line is that advertising to children is exploitative, affecting both children's product purchase requests and parents' purchasing decisions.

WORK, SCHOOL, AND THE BUILT ENVIRONMENT

Another major change in the modern world, besides the foods we eat, is that many people are less physically active than people were in the past. Many factors have contributed to this decline in physical activity, including changes in workplaces, schools, and the built environment in general.

One contributor to our increasingly sedentary lifestyles is a changing labor market.[12] In 1950, 30 percent of adults in the United States worked in jobs that involved high levels of physical activity, such as construction, farming, or restaurant work. By 2000, only 22 percent worked in such occupations. In contrast, the percentage of people working in low-activity jobs, such as office jobs or trucking, rose from roughly 23 percent to 41 percent over this period. With the industrialization of agriculture, fewer Americans needed to do hard-labor jobs on farms. Instead, many migrated to urban environments and transitioned into more sedentary office or service-based work. In addition, technological innovations have caused people to spend more and more time on their phones and computers, or watching television than ever before, time that is generally devoid of physical activity.

Beyond their effects on physical activity, workplace environments promote obesity in other ways. Many offices supply unhealthy sugary drinks and snacks to workers, which encourages them to consume more, ostensibly to sustain or increase their energy levels. Many workplaces also provide vending machines with high-calorie snacks and drinks and few healthy options. The design of the modern workplace prioritizes close parking, relies on elevators rather than stairs, and provides few facilities for exercise. Workplace environments can create job stress and chronic fatigue, both of which are associated with poor diets, reduced physical activity, and an increased risk of obesity. Shift workers and employees who work longer-than-usual hours every week, for example, have a higher risk of obesity.[13]

Just as adults in the United States spend more than one-quarter of all their time at work, children spend much of their day at school, and schools often promote unhealthy eating habits and sedentary behaviors. The National School Lunch Program and related federal school meal programs, which every school day serve more than 30 million children breakfasts, lunches, and after-school snacks, have not been shown to increase the risk of obesity, but most schools also sell "junk foods" to students outside of these school meal programs. These foods with low nutrition values are readily available in cafeterias, vending machines, and school stores, and schools often offer sugar-sweetened beverages. Although recent agreements between the Alliance for a Healthier Generation and the American Beverage Association have significantly reduced the amount of sugar-sweetened beverages sold in schools, this problem is far from being eliminated. Furthermore, when the No Child Left Behind Act went into effect in the United States, many schools cut recess and physical education periods to allow for longer classes in order to meet the higher standards for reading and math. In recent years, some states have begun to implement recess laws and physical education standards. Hopefully, more states will follow suit as the long-lasting benefits to children of physical activity become more widely known.

The built environment in general has contributed to the increase in obesity rates. Urban environments may favor roads over pedestrian and bike paths, may lack parks and sidewalks, and may be unsafe for children to play outside. Again, this is particularly true in poorer neighborhoods. Problems in neighborhoods can range from reckless drivers to narcotic and criminal activities to bullies on the playground. If people believe that their neighborhoods are unsafe, children will be less likely to play outside and adults will be reluctant to walk or take part in other physical activities.[14] In contrast, people who live in areas that they trust, in which they feel safe, and that foster social cohesion typically have higher levels of physical activity and therefore a better chance of protecting themselves against weight gain.

THE HOME ENVIRONMENT

Cultural norms and practices around eating are first learned in the homes where we grow up. Our parents, grandparents, and guardians model eating habits and set up structures within the household around snacking and meals. Some families eat multiple meals together; others don't share a single meal in the day. Some parents force their children to "clean their plates"; some allow their children to stop eating when they're full. Some parents accommodate their children's picky preferences; others insist that they try new foods. With all the different ways in which families influence a child's eating habits, separating out the factors that contribute to obesity is difficult.

Unsurprisingly, there is a strong connection between the availability of fruits and vegetables at home and whether children, adolescents, and adults eat these foods.[15] Eating meals as a family has also been associated with greater consumption of fruits, vegetables, and other healthy foods among both children and adults.[16] Unfortunately, the frequency of family dinners has declined over the past 20 years, with the majority of American families eating a meal together less than five days a week. This is especially concerning in light of research that shows that children who do not eat dinner with their parents at least twice a week are 40 percent more likely to be overweight compared with those who do.[17] Eating together as a family, beyond the psychological benefits, is one way in which parents can model and support healthy eating habits and may be a strategy to protect against overweight and obesity.

Two feeding practices that researchers have studied in the past are parental restriction and pressure to eat. Many of these studies have been based around the assumption that highly controlled feeding practices, such as requiring a child to clean their plate, bribing a child to eat, or restricting access to palatable foods, lead children to focus more on external cues rather than internal cues in determining whether they have eaten enough. External cues might be parent demands, food characteristics, and food left on the plate, while internal cues include feelings of hunger and fullness. These studies have suggested that highly controlled feeding practices, compounded with increasingly obesogenic environments, cause children who are fed in this way to eat more in the absence of hunger or to continue eating even when they're full.[18]

Recently, researchers have broadened the scope of their work to examine overall household feeding styles. A feeding style refers to the overall attitude and emotional climate that a parent establishes with a child with regard to eating. Feeding styles are measured along two dimensions: parental demandingness and responsiveness, with demandingness referring to the number of demands that parents place on a child to eat, and responsiveness referring to how sensitive parents are to a child's eating needs and preferences. Four different parenting styles exist along this spectrum.[19] An authoritative style, in which parents exhibit high demandingness and high responsiveness, tends to be the most conducive toward healthy eating behaviors, with parents placing reasonable nutritional demands on their child as well as being sensitive to the child's needs. Authoritarian parents, who have high demands and low responsiveness, tend to have less success as they are highly controlling during feeding episodes and show little sensitivity toward the child. Indulgent parents, who exhibit low demandingness and high responsiveness, are also less effective at promoting healthy eating behaviors. Though they are highly responsive to their child's needs, they provide few rules and little structure that gives the child the freedom to determine their own nutritional intake. Finally, uninvolved parents who exhibit low demandingness and low responsiveness are also ineffective at encouraging healthy choices as they demonstrate little control and involvement during feeding.

Again, low-income families fare significantly worse in being able to foster healthy home environments. Healthy foods such as fruits, vegetables, and whole grains tend to be more expensive than unhealthy foods such as refined grains and sweets and therefore may be prohibitively expensive for low-income families. In addition, healthful meals often require preparation, whereas convenience or fast food is by definition ready almost instantly.

EATING OUT VERSUS EATING AT HOME

Higher rates of obesity are related to the shift from home-cooked meals to eating out. The prevalence of eating out significantly increased at the beginning of the 1970s, shortly before the start of the obesity epidemic. In 2014, for the first time since the Commerce Department started tracking US spending habits on food in 1992, Americans spent more money at restaurants and bars than at grocery stores. A recent study reported that more than one in three Americans eats at least one fast food meal every single day; in 2012 the average American ate more than two hundred meals outside the home.[20]

Even as people began eating more meals away from home, portion sizes of food and drink grew dramatically. The portions served in restaurants are double or triple what they used to be, mostly because ingredients are cheaper and costs are low. Studies show that when people are served larger portions, they eat more with no decrease in later food consumption.[21] In one study, subjects were given macaroni and cheese in various portion sizes. The bigger the portion size, the more the participants ate.[22]

There are many reasons why people are eating out more than ever before. Throughout the twentieth century, two-income households became increasingly common as more women entered the workforce. Consequently, women had less time to cook, which drove demand for quick and convenient meals. In addition, two-income households had more money to spend on food, potentially making it easier to justify meals away from the home, especially with both parents working most of the day.

The increase in divorce rates and single-parent households has also contributed to the growing desire for fast, tasty, and convenient meals. In single-parent households, parents often have to work long hours to make ends meet, leaving them little time or energy to shop for, prepare, and cook fresh, healthy meals. Lower incomes and higher instability related to living transitions may pose further challenges to promoting healthy eating behaviors in single-parent households. A recent study supported these hypotheses, finding higher BMIs and obesogenic behaviors in children of single-parent households.[23]

A CHANGING RELATIONSHIP WITH FOOD

In the past couple of decades, people are spending more time than ever using mobile devices and watching TV in their homes. Unfortunately, numerous studies have shown that the more television people watch, the more likely they are to gain weight or become overweight or obese.[24] Perhaps the association reflects a tendency to snack while watching TV or interacting with online media; perhaps it reflects a disruption of normal meals or a simple lack of physical activity. While screen time does not in itself contribute to weight gain, it's a marker of our increasingly sedentary lifestyles and our changing relationship with food.

Mindlessly eating while watching TV or playing video games is part of a larger shift toward grazing, or the repetitive act of eating small amounts of food throughout the day rather than eating three normal meals. Though some Americans still eat breakfast, lunch, and dinner, most Americans snack between meals and often do not view these snacks as a significant source of calories. There's nothing wrong with snacking when hungry in order to last until the next meal; what sets grazing apart is the frequency with which snacking occurs and the fact that it happens regardless of hunger or satiety sensations. One study found that grazing was a clinically significant form of overeating associated with binge eating, weight gain, and reduced treatment success for obesity.[25] When I see patients who want to lose weight, I frequently advise them to start a daily food journal and also to take photos of everything they eat. Often when they return for their next visit, they report being shocked at the amounts of foods consumed outside of breakfast, lunch, and dinner.

Our society places a major emphasis on social eating. Bars, restaurants, convenience stores, and fast-food outlets are everywhere and serve as meeting places for many social gatherings. Food has always been a way of connecting, of spreading love, and of relaxing. It's wonderful to share a good meal with family and friends. But the cultural role that food plays in our society can distance hunger from eating, which can promote overeating, mindless eating, and indulgent eating.

In addition to working longer hours for less pay to meet economic needs, many new stressors have emerged in our modern landscape that significantly affect our behaviors. Poor interpersonal relationships, job or unemployment stress, low self-esteem, and low socioeconomic status can all lead to chronic social stress—persistent stress regarding one's social environment—which is linked to obesity and its associated illnesses. In particular, a recent study has shown that increased long-term levels of cortisol in our blood (which reflect long-term stress) drive appetite and cravings and are strongly related to abdominal obesity, insulin resistance, diabetes, and cardiovascular diseases.[26] Stress promotes cravings for nutrient-dense "comfort foods."[27] These altered feeding behaviors may cause weight gain, which may result in additional stress, and the cycle begins again. Research reports found that among individuals with obesity, roughly half exhibit cortisol levels within the normal range, while the other half exhibit higher cortisol levels. Elevated cortisol levels, indicative of stress, predispose individuals toward obesity.

Poor sleep habits are also contributing to the obesity crisis. According to one study involving 440,000 people, more than a third of US adults are getting less than seven hours of sleep per night.[28] Too little sleep increases the risk for many serious health conditions, including obesity, diabetes, high blood pressure, heart disease, stroke, and frequent mental distress. According to the Nurses' Health Study, which followed 68,000 middle-aged American women for up to 16 years, women who slept five hours or less were 15 percent more likely to become obese over the course of the study than women who slept seven hours a night.[29]

Why is sleep so important? Sleep deprivation may alter the hormones that control hunger. Furthermore, people who sleep less each night have more waking time to eat. Sleep deprivation makes it more difficult to resist temptation, thereby encouraging people to choose less healthy foods. It can also increase the tendency to go out to eat, to have irregular meal patterns, and to snack more than those who get adequate sleep. Sleep deprivation makes you more tired during the day, resulting in curbed physical activity. Finally, people who are sleep deprived may experience a drop in their body temperatures associated with decreased energy expenditure.

DEFECTS IN THE CONTROL OF EATING

Overeating can also result from hedonic hunger, which can be defined as a desire to eat even in the absence of an energy deficit. This desire doesn't arise from biological hunger; rather, it comes from the anticipated pleasure of eating. In a society filled with convenient, cheap, and energy-dense foods, hedonic eating can override the other controls on what we eat, altering the body's ability to regulate its consumption of food.

Hedonic eating occurs along a spectrum. At one end of the spectrum is a situation such as being present at a dinner with friends. People might eat and drink to excess not because they're hungry but as a result of their food environment. At the other end of the spectrum is a situation such as binging on junk food in front of the TV. In this instance, an emotional trigger drives the desire to replace negative feelings with pleasurable rewards. An endless onslaught of food and beverage advertisements, options, and pressures to eat has distanced us from listening to our body's hunger cues. In modern society, there are few environments that don't encourage hedonic eating.

Ruth complained about episodes of "losing control over her eating." Affecting about 3 percent of American adults in their lifetime, binge eating disorder (BED) is characterized by frequently consuming unusually large amounts of food in one sitting and feeling that one's eating behavior is out of control.[30] Studies suggest that nearly half the risk for developing BED is genetic.[31] Nearly half of BED patients have a comorbid mood disorder, and more than half of BED patients have comorbid anxiety disorders. However, while these conditions are clearly influenced by genetics, environmental structures also contribute to their development because they provide the access, cues, and stressors that promote food addiction and BED.

Bulimia differs from BED by involving not only excessive eating but purging food through vomiting, inducing diarrhea, or excessive exercising in an attempt to lose weight. Bulimia can be cyclical, disappearing for periods and then recurring. Both BED and bulimia have diagnostic criteria that allow for diagnoses and treatment.

A more controversial condition is known as "food addiction." In such cases, people are triggered to eat by cues associated with palatable foods. Some food addiction theories point to neurobiological studies that identify shared brain mechanisms that occur when eating and taking recreational drugs or other addictive behaviors. However, focusing only on the similarities between the brain mechanisms for overeating and addiction ignores the fact that food is essential for survival, whereas other pleasurable and addictive behaviors are not.

Much more research will need to be done to understand the ways in which eating disorders occur and how they relate to weight gain. In particular, studies need to examine how hedonic eating influences the body, how we respond to food-associated external cues, and how we develop impaired inhibitory control over food cravings.

SWIMMING AGAINST THE TIDE

An overwhelming variety of forces over the past half century have caused people to overeat and gain weight. Furthermore, as these forces become more powerful and widespread, more people are susceptible to them. Our societies and environments are full of incentives to overeat and minimize physical activity.

Reversing the damage that has been done by these incentives will require both individual and societal action, as described in chapters 4 and 5 of this book. But before looking at what is needed, we need to consider obesity's effects on health.

CHAPTER 3

What Are the Consequences of Obesity?

THE EFFECTS OF OBESITY ON health are well known, including a higher risk of developing diabetes, high blood pressure, coronary artery disease, stroke, and other diseases. The psychological consequences of obesity are cited less often, but they, too, can be severe, chronic, and debilitating. In this chapter, I'll start with these psychological consequences before moving on to physical health conditions.

CHANGING PERCEPTIONS

In the past, being plump wasn't stigmatized the way it is today. Earth goddess sculptures from 25,000 years ago depicted round women as objects of beauty and fertility. During the Renaissance, being "Rubenesque" was a desirable trait that signified power and wealth, because rich people could afford plentiful food while the poor could not. Obesity is still associated with wealth, beauty, good health, strength, and respect in some parts of the world.

But this dynamic has been changing worldwide. Due to the

rising availability, accessibility, and affordability of fast foods and processed foods, poor people can afford high-calorie, lower-nutrient foods, raising their likelihood of becoming overweight or obese. Wealthier individuals can afford healthier foods, making them more likely to be thin. As a result, people today are more prone to associate thinness with both wealth and health. Western diets are not the only thing that has spread throughout the world—so have ideas about which bodies are beautiful.

Today, many people see obesity as the result of overindulgence, laziness, and a lack of willpower. This seems especially unfair given how we judge other medical conditions. We don't blame people with high cholesterol or high blood pressure for their conditions. Yet people with excess weight are regularly accused of bringing the condition upon themselves. Furthermore, the visibility of obesity makes it different from other conditions. Few medical conditions can be diagnosed as soon as a patient walks through the door. The conspicuousness of obesity places a huge psychological burden on those with excess weight.

Science has made great advances in understanding the biological underpinnings of obesity. Much less progress has been made in understanding the cultural dimensions of this chronic and complex condition.

STIGMA AND PREJUDICE

While discussing other differences between people has become taboo, fat shaming has remained a common form of ridicule.

Movies often poke fun at people with obesity, the message being that if you're not a "normal" size you're somehow worth less than other people. Television sitcoms frequently use bodies of characters who are overweight as the butt of jokes. Even greeting or birthday cards often display "funny" photos of fat people.

Although parents and friends may believe that shame is motivational, using shame as a parenting and teaching technique has been consistently shown to result in negative outcomes for children. Furthermore, shame implies an internal failure, and obesity results from much more than personal weakness. Children whose parents use shame to motivate behavioral change often suffer from low self-esteem and are at higher risk for mental disorders including anxiety, depression, obsessive compulsive disorder, and eating disorders.[1] In adults, consistent shaming about weight, a factor that often feels out of a person's control, similarly appears harmful rather than motivating, often resulting in the opposite of the intended effects.

Perhaps the most prominent form of fat shaming exists on social media and the internet. Online trolls are constantly degrading and insulting individuals for their weight and appearance. This fat shaming tends to be targeted at women, and even those who are only marginally overweight are often victims of such abuse. When celebrities successfully lose weight, they're praised for their efforts; when the weight creeps back on, they're mocked for failing.

America has become obsessed with thinness—but not because of its relation to health. Instead, thinness has become the ultimate aesthetic ideal, a symbol of hard work, self-control, and determination. In a study of 4,283 people that included representation across the weight spectrum, 46 percent of respondents reported that they would be willing to give up at least one year of life rather than be obese, 15 percent reported that they would be willing to give up 10 years or more of their life, 25 percent reported that they would rather be unable to have children than to be obese, 15 percent reported that they would rather be severely depressed, and 14 percent reported that they would rather be alcoholic.[2] Let these numbers sink in.

This obsession with thinness has contributed to a rapid increase in eating disorders, especially among young women. Today, roughly 30 million people struggle with eating disorders in the United States, a significant number of whom are also obese.[3] This fixation on thinness and disgust with fatness even appears to have an effect on mortality. A 2015 study found that people who reported experiencing weight discrimination had a 60 percent increased risk of dying, regardless of size.[4]

Widespread negative stereotypes around obesity drive the common belief that a person's weight is entirely the individual's responsibility. These stereotypes also affect the interactions that people who are overweight have with loved ones, family members, friends, coworkers, and strangers. Studies have shown that people with obesity earn less than their peers, are passed over for job promotions more frequently than normal-weight people, and are consistently discriminated against in the workplace. More than 40 percent of Americans with obesity report experiencing stigma on a daily basis.[5]

Dealing with such a constant onslaught of negative stereotypes can affect your perceptions and ideas about yourself. People with obesity often stigmatize themselves, blaming themselves for being fat in the same way that others do, whereas many other stigmatized groups come together to support one another in the face of prejudice.

Fat shaming starts early, with weight being one of the most common reasons that children are bullied in school. In one study, 84 percent of students reported observing their peers who are overweight being teased and bullied during physical activities.[6] The same study found that 65 to 77 percent of students observed peers with overweight or obesity being ignored, avoided, excluded from social activities, having negative rumors spread about them, and being teased in the cafeteria.

Women also tend to bear more weight-based victimization at lighter relative weights than their male counterparts. Women tend to experience weight-based bullying when they are in the overweight range, while for men body shaming tends to become a factor only when they are obese. Women who are obese report three times as much body-shaming and weight-based discrimination than do men with the same level of obesity.[7]

Even corporations often resort to fat shaming. Purported "corporate wellness" programs may overemphasize incentivizing weight loss through monetary reward. Some employers use programs in which employees are divided into teams that compete against one another to lose the most weight. These "games," which often last for several months, can encourage disordered eating and drastic weight loss tactics while also shaming those who struggle to lose weight. Furthermore, in most cases these programs don't achieve the weight loss goal and don't save employers money.[8] Employee weight loss often does not generate lower health care spending or higher productivity because, most of the time, employees gain the weight back.

Contending with constant external and internal judgments about their self-worth is one reason why people with overweight and obesity have higher rates of anxiety, depression, low self-esteem, eating disorders, and exercise avoidance. Furthermore, experiencing the shame and stress that comes with fat shaming can trigger biological processes that drive some to overeat and gain more weight. When people are stressed, a hormone called cortisol is released, which can stimulate appetite, increase the accumulation of belly fat, and increase the risks for diabetes and depression. It's a vicious cycle of stress, weight gain, and poor health.

Furthermore, it appears that the relationship between depression and obesity may be bidirectional, with depression raising the risk for developing obesity and obesity raising the risk for developing depression.[9] Although a biological link has yet to be definitively identified, possible mechanisms related to the development of depression in people with obesity include changes in brain chemistry, inflammation, and hormone levels, compounded by social and cultural factors.

FIGHTING BACK AGAINST STIGMA

Despite the continued prevalence of weight-based stereotyping and fat shaming in American culture, the discourse has been changing. Widespread public support has resulted in anti-bullying laws that include protection for children who are overweight and laws that prohibit discrimination against obesity in the workplace. The past several years have also seen a rise in the body positive movement, a social movement rooted in the belief that all people should have a positive body image no matter their appearance. This movement gained popularity in the early 2010s, with an initial focus on the unrealistic feminine beauty standards portrayed in the media and across consumer spaces. As more and more people joined the movement, the message expanded to "All bodies are beautiful." Over time, product brands and influencers have taken up the trend. Events such as Curvy Con, an annual convention celebrating plus-size brands and individuals, and media such as "Fattitude," a film about weight stigma, are helping to raise greater awareness of weight biases.

One spokesperson for the body positive movement is the singer, rapper, songwriter, and flutist Lizzo. She faces immense online trolling and comments about her weight. In response to a recent critique about her size, Lizzo responded that she has been working out regularly for the past five years but that she does it for herself. She said that she is not aiming for the ideal body type but for *her* ideal body type. "Health is not just what you look like on the outside," she said. "Health is also what happens on the inside." I couldn't agree more, and I'll have a lot more to say about this issue in chapter 4.

DIABETES, CARDIOVASCULAR DISEASE, AND METABOLIC SYNDROME

Being obese does not guarantee that someone will develop a disease associated with obesity, but it increases the risk. Furthermore, this risk is heightened in older people, in racial and ethnic minorities, and in some immigrant groups in the United States.[10]

The correlation between obesity and type 2 diabetes is stronger than for other comorbidities.[11] One reason for this relationship is that fat cells in the abdomen secrete hormones and other substances that cause inflammation, cellular stress, and insulin resistance. Although inflammation is an essential part of the immune response and healing process, chronic inflammation can result in a variety of health problems. Most importantly, inflammation can cause the body to be less responsive to insulin, the hormone related to the development of diabetes.

The more overweight you are, the more insulin you make.

That's because, as you gain weight, the beta cells in the pancreas that make insulin try to compensate for the excess fat storage in the body by enlarging and by producing and releasing more insulin. But continued demand on the insulin production system can cause it to falter and then fail. Eventually, cells that make insulin no longer respond appropriately to nutrients and hormonal signals. When this happens, a person develops type 2 diabetes, characterized by persistently elevated blood glucose levels.

Two large epidemiological studies found that the risk for type 2 diabetes begins to increase at the overweight BMI levels (25–30). It then increases more steeply when BMI exceeds 30.[12] Compared with men and women with BMIs below 25, men with BMIs of 30 or higher have a sevenfold greater risk of developing type 2 diabetes, and women with BMIs of 30 or higher have a twelvefold greater risk.[13] Risk also varies among racial and ethnic groups, with Native Americans, African Americans, Mexican Americans, Pacific Islander, and South Asian populations at greater risk for type 2 diabetes than whites, due to genetic as well as environmental differences.

Obesity is also a major risk factor for cardiovascular disease. As BMI increases, so do blood pressure, low-density lipoprotein cholesterol (or "bad cholesterol"), triglycerides, blood sugar, and inflammation. High-density lipoprotein cholesterol (so-called good cholesterol) decreases with obesity. These factors all increase the risk for coronary heart disease, stroke, and cardiovascular death. As with the development of type 2 diabetes, the relationship between weight and the risk of cardiovascular disease varies among racial and ethnic groups. African Americans may have less risk at a given BMI than whites, while persons of Asian descent might be at the most risk, due to genetic differences in fat distribution and lipid metabolism. Across all populations, cardiovascular disease is the main cause of death in obesity relative to people of normal weights. The more overweight you are, the more likely you are to die from a heart attack, both for men and women.

A broader problem is the metabolic syndrome I described in chapter 1, a condition defined by abdominal obesity, increased blood pressure, elevated glucose and triglyceride levels, and low levels of beneficial high-density cholesterol. The prevalence of metabolic syndrome has increased globally, primarily due to excessive intake of energy-dense foods, reduced physical activity, low socioeconomic status, and rapid urbanization. As with obesity, metabolic syndrome increases the risk of developing cardiovascular diseases, nonalcoholic fatty liver disease, cancer, infertility, dementia, and other diseases. In the United States, one study found that more than 80 percent of participants age 50 years or older with diabetes also had metabolic syndrome.[14]

THE REPRODUCTIVE SYSTEM

Obesity can also adversely impact various aspects of reproduction, from sexual activity to conception. Part of this stems from the fact that adipose tissues help control the levels and potency of sex hormones. For women, infertility is lowest among women with normal BMI and increases with both lower and higher BMIs.

Part of the reason why heavy women have more difficulty conceiving relates to dysregulation of the sex hormones that regulate ovulation.[15] Being obese during pregnancy also heightens the risk of problems, including miscarriage, new-onset (gestational) diabetes, preeclampsia (high blood pressure and protein leak in the urine), and complications during labor and delivery. Furthermore, as with depression, infertility and extra weight may have a bidirectional relationship. Attempting to become pregnant, especially if it is difficult, may result in elevated stress, which may drive stress eating that further harms fertility.

Reduced fertility has similarly been shown among men who are obese, though the evidence is less clear. A 2012 study showed that men with obesity are more likely to have low sperm counts.[16] For one thing, obesity can elevate body temperature around the scrotum, which may be harmful to sperm production. Also, obesity can lead to hormonal imbalances; men with obesity are more likely to have higher estrogen levels combined with lower levels of testosterone. Together, these factors can affect sperm production and the ability of sperm to swim well.[17] Studies have also shown that the odds of developing erectile dysfunction increase with increasing BMI.[18]

THE LIVER AND LUNGS

────────

Another potential consequence of obesity is nonalcoholic fatty liver disease (NAFLD) and nonalcoholic steatohepatitis. Experts suggest that between 30 and 40 percent of American adults have some degree of NAFLD, making it the most common chronic liver condition in the United States. The less serious form of NAFLD is characterized by excessive fat accumulation in the liver but little or no inflammation of the liver or damage to liver cells, and this form of NAFLD generally does not progress to liver damage. However, among adults with NAFLD in the United States, roughly 20 percent have the more serious form of NAFLD called nonalcoholic steatohepatitis (NASH), representing between 3 percent and 12 percent of the US adult population.[19] NASH causes hepatitis—inflammation of the liver—as well as damage to liver cells. Inflammation paired with liver cell damage can progress to fibrosis, in which the liver's connective tissue is thickened or scarred, and cirrhosis, where hard scar tissue replaces an increasingly larger amount of healthy liver tissue. Approximately 5 percent of patients with obesity develop cirrhosis, though further studies are needed to determine why some people and not others develop these conditions.

Obesity can also compromise lung function and increase the risk of developing respiratory disease. Larger stores of abdominal fat may prevent the diaphragm from descending properly, restricting lung expansion. At the same time, the accumulation of fat can reduce the flexibility of the chest wall, decreasing respiratory muscle strength and narrowing the airways in the lungs. A low-grade inflammatory state caused by obesity may further impair lung function.

Obesity is associated with greater risk of asthma and obstructive sleep apnea. Obstructive sleep apnea causes breathing to repeatedly stop and start during sleep. This condition affects roughly one in five adults, and between half and three-quarters of those affected are obese.[20] Obstructive sleep apnea is associated with daytime sleepiness, high blood pressure, cardiovascular disease, and premature death.

DEMENTIA

Many studies have associated obesity during middle age with a higher risk of dementia later in life.[21] However, the relationship, as with so many other aspects of obesity, is complex. BMI does not seem to be a factor in the cognitive function of older adults, but a measure of central obesity, the waist-to-hip ratio, is linked to cognitive decline.[22] Furthermore, this measure of central obesity has been linked to a higher risk of developing late-onset Alzheimer's disease.[23]

People who have a high BMI and central obesity are at the greatest risk for dementia (3.5 times increased risk). People with a healthy BMI who are centrally obese still have roughly double the risk for developing dementia compared with people who do not have excess belly fat.[24] These associations may relate to the finding that otherwise healthy middle-aged adults with central obesity tend to have smaller brain volumes, suggesting possible brain shrinkage.[25]

The link between obesity and dementia might relate to the impact of fat hormones (adipokines), insulin resistance, and inflammation on the brain. Until recently, it was thought that systemic inflammation predisposes individuals to diabetes by disrupting the functions of liver and muscle but not the brain. However, many mediators of systemic inflammation do cross the blood-brain barrier. Also, metabolic mediators released by adipose tissue and other organs play important roles in brain health. It may be that a cycle is created in which neurons are exposed to injury because of inflammation and metabolic stress, which sets up a cascade of neurodegeneration. Taken together, these studies indicate that maintaining a healthy body weight could prevent, or at least delay, the development of dementia.

CANCER

The relationship between body weight and cancer is also complex, in part because cancer is not a single disease but a collection of individual diseases. However, many studies have linked obesity to increased risk of certain types of cancer.[26] Consistent evidence shows that higher amounts of body fat are associated with higher risks of breast cancer, endometrial cancer (cancer of the lining of the uterus), esophageal adenocarcinoma (cancer of the esophagus), gastric cardia cancer (cancer in the upper part of the stomach), liver cancer, kidney cancer, multiple myeloma (cancer of the plasma cells), meningioma (a slow-growing tumor of the outer covering of the brain), pancreatic cancer, colorectal cancer, gall bladder cancer, and ovarian cancer.

A 2012 population-based study that examined BMI and cancer incidence in the United States found that about 28,000 new cases of cancer in men (3.5 percent of the total) and 72,000 in women (9.5 percent) were attributable to overweight or obesity.[27] However, the relationship was as high as 54 percent for gallbladder cancer in women and 44 percent for esophageal adenocarcinoma in men. A 2016 study that compared cancer and obesity rates among countries found that the United States had the highest rates of colorectal cancer, pancreatic cancer, and postmenopausal breast cancer caused by overweight or obesity.[28]

Several hypotheses seek to account for the association between obesity and these types of cancers. Chronic inflammation may cause DNA damage that promotes cancer. Adipose tissue produces excess amounts of estrogen and alters the levels of fat hormones (adipokines), which are associated with an increased risk of breast, endometrial, ovarian, and some other cancers. People with obesity also tend to have high levels of insulin and insulin-like growth factor, which may promote the development of colon, kidney, prostate, and endometrial cancers.

MUSCULOSKELETAL DISORDERS

Obesity can result in musculoskeletal disorders, including both degenerative and inflammatory conditions. Osteoarthritis is the most common type of arthritis, and today rates are higher than ever, likely driven by the obesity epidemic.

Studies have consistently shown that the more you weigh, the greater your risk of developing osteoarthritis in large joints. The condition occurs when the cartilage that cushions and protects the ends of bones in joints wears down over time, causing pain, decreased mobility, and lower quality of life. Added weight puts more pressure and stress on weight-bearing joints, which makes heavier people particularly vulnerable to osteoarthritis of the knee and the hip. Women with obesity, for example, have a nearly fourfold greater risk of knee osteoarthritis than women who are not obese, and men with obesity have a nearly fivefold greater risk.[29] Osteoarthritis also progresses more quickly and is more severe among people with obesity than among people who weigh less. Consequentially, patients with obesity account for one-third of all joint replacement operations.[30] Obesity also raises the risk of back pain, lower limb pain, and disability due to musculoskeletal conditions related to bearing the load of excess weight.

Weight loss can substantially improve the prognosis for those with arthritis. It can lead to reduced joint pain and inflammation, better joint function, lower risk of comorbid conditions, more energy, and sounder sleep. This makes sense when you realize that every pound of excess weight exerts three to six pounds of extra force on the joints. Thus if you're 100 pounds overweight, you're putting an extra 300 to 600 extra pounds of pressure on your joints with every step.[31] Losing even 10 pounds will result in 30 pounds less pressure per knee per step. For a person who walks 5,000 steps per day, this adds up to nearly 55 million less pounds of pressure on the knees each year.

CHILDHOOD OBESITY

The World Health Organization (WHO) has called childhood obesity "one of the most serious public health challenges of the 21st century."[32] The WHO is right. Obesity can damage almost every system in a child's body. It can wreak havoc on blood sugar control, the heart, the lungs, the muscles and bones, the kidneys, and the digestive tract. It can disrupt the hormones that control puberty, resulting in a serious social and emotional toll. Furthermore, studies have found that youth who are overweight or obese have significantly higher odds of remaining overweight or obese into adulthood, further increasing their risk of disease and disability later in life.[33]

Globally, 38 million children under the age of 5 were overweight or obese in 2019.[34] In 2016, more than 340 million children and adolescents ages 5 to 19 were overweight or obese. Childhood obesity rates are rising everywhere, but increases have been particularly alarming in many low-income countries. In Africa, the number of children under 5 who are overweight has grown by nearly 24 percent since 2000.

The rise in childhood obesity rates occurred simultaneously with the rise in adult obesity rates, with the sharpest increases occurring during the 1980s and 1990s. In 1975, only 4 percent of all children and adolescents ages 5 to 19 were overweight or obese. By 2016, 18 percent of this age group was overweight or obese, with similar increases among both boys and girls. Recently, the greatest increases in obesity have occurred among children ages 2 to 5, which is particularly worrisome since obesity at this age predisposes children to obesity in adulthood and lifelong health problems.

Childhood obesity affects children in both richer and poorer countries, but the contributors to obesity appear to differ somewhat among nations. In the United States and other wealthy countries, toxic food environments and inactivity appear to be the largest drivers of childhood obesity. However, awareness of the dangers of sugar and soda consumption has increased, and restricted access may make these products less of a contributing factor than they once were. On the other hand, in countries such as China, India, and Brazil, many children still consume large amounts of sugar and soda, especially in areas where water is not drinkable. Children in these countries are also facing the "nutrition transition," which describes a shift toward more Western dietary patterns marked by increased consumption of red meat, processed foods, and fast foods. The increased availability of these products has improved food security in many cases, but it has also had negative health consequences.

RISK FACTORS DURING FETAL DEVELOPMENT

The origins of childhood obesity begin well before a child is born. In the womb, the physiological systems providing nutrients and oxygen to the fetus function differently depending on a mother's health. For instance, if a mother is obese and diabetic, then her child is more likely to be born obese and to later become diabetic.

Four factors appear to play the biggest roles in predisposing children in the womb to later obesity: the mother's smoking habits during pregnancy, the mother's weight gain during pregnancy, the mother's obesity status prior to and during pregnancy, and the mother's blood sugar levels during pregnancy, specifically if she develops pregnancy-related diabetes. However, assessing the role of these factors is difficult, because mothers with extra weight are also more likely to provide obesogenic environments to their offspring.

Once a child is born, parental influences can further promote the development of obesity. How rapidly an infant gains weight, how long an infant is breastfed, and how much an infant sleeps can all influence weight gain later in life. Accelerated weight gain during the first weeks or months of an infant's life is associated with higher BMI or obesity later in life. Whether breastfeeding can protect against obesity may be debatable, but some studies have shown that the longer a mother breastfeeds her child, the lower her child's chance of developing obesity later in life.

HEALTH CONSEQUENCES IN CHILDREN

Tragically, type 2 diabetes, NAFLD, and cardiovascular diseases, once thought to occur only in adults, are now seen among children with obesity. Especially worrisome is the fact that type 2 diabetes tends to be more aggressive in children than it is in adults. Children with higher BMIs also tend to have higher blood pressure and lipid levels, factors that increase cardiovascular risk among adults. A study of nearly 2.3 million people who were followed over the course of 40 years found that the risk of dying from heart disease was two to three times greater if they had been overweight or obese as teenagers.[35]

Weight-related concerns also impact children's mental health. Nearly half of 3- to 6-year-old girls report worrying about being fat.[36] Perhaps this is appropriate, since the health-related quality of life among children and adolescents with obesity has been shown to be substantially lower than among their non-obese counterparts. Sadly, the quality-of-life scores for children with severe obesity were similar to those among children with cancers.[37]

The stage for excess weight gain is clearly set early in life. Children depend on parents and elders to guide their eating behaviors. Children are also more susceptible to outside influences like food and beverage marketing. Blaming children for being obese reveals the hypocrisy of blaming anyone for their obesity. Children do not get to decide their weight. They need healthier environments and influences to counter the genetic and environmental factors that contribute to their extra weight.

THE OBESITY-MORTALITY PARADOX

As I have emphasized, obesity is a major risk factor for developing serious diseases. At the same time, some studies have shown that being overweight may be beneficial under some circumstances. For example, being overweight may speed recovery time from illness. When you're sick, your body may require more energy to heal properly. To some extent, excess fat may provide this crucial source for recovery. Furthermore, older people have less of a connection between weight and mortality than do younger people. Perhaps by old age the benefits of extra weight outweigh the negative effects.

The so-called obesity-mortality paradox rose to public attention after studies found reduced mortality rates among people with overweight and obesity who had heart failure, terminal cancer, coronary vascular disease, kidney failure, and other chronic wasting diseases. For example, the Atherosclerosis Risk in Communities study investigated 1,279 individuals and found that among patients hospitalized with a diagnosis of heart failure, mortality was higher in normal-weight individuals than in the people with overweight.[38] Similarly, a large study of 345,192 patients from the British Cardiovascular Intervention Society registry revealed that people with higher BMIs who underwent a procedure to treat the narrowing of blood vessels had lower mortality than did thinner people.[39]

The relationship between excess weight and mortality received further notice after a 2013 study that examined mortality and obesity among nearly 3 million people.[40] The study divided participants into four groups: those with a relatively normal BMI between 18.5 and 25 (a healthy BMI), those with a BMI between 25 and 30 (who are conventionally defined as overweight), those with BMIs between 30 and 35 (defined as grade 1 obese), and those with BMIs above 35 (defined as grades 2 and 3 obesity). In comparison with normal-weight participants, the participants who were obese in general and those with grades 2 and 3 obesity had significantly greater all-cause mortality. However, participants with grade 1 obesity did not have higher mortality rates, and people who were merely overweight had significantly reduced rates of mortality. These findings suggested that being overweight had a protective influence on health and that mild obesity was not harmful.

These results have fueled arguments ever since they were released. The studies have been critiqued for their design and conclusions, such as not adequately adjusting for weight loss and higher mortality from chronic illnesses, smoking, and aging. Such arguments spurred researchers to attempt to identify possible sources of bias or confounding variables that might have distorted the conclusions. For instance, if smokers or patients with severe chronic diseases such as cancer (groups with lower average BMIs but very high mortality risk) are included in the at-risk population, these factors could have caused a false association between lower-weight people and death. These studies might also create a situation of reverse causation, in which the direction of cause and effect is contrary to the presumed relationship between weight and mortality. As a result of these concerns, several other large studies have demonstrated that when smokers and those with known cancers are excluded from the data analysis, mortality increases in a linear manner for participants with overweight, obesity, and severe obesity.[41]

At the same time, other studies that account for confounding factors do not resolve the obesity paradox.[42] For instance, one looked at the association between BMI and mortality in newly diagnosed diabetic patients in the United States and found that deaths from all causes, from cardiovascular diseases, and from other diseases were higher for normal BMI participants than for those with overweight or obese BMIs.[43] In another 15-year study of African American and Caucasian male veterans with diabetes, BMI was again inversely associated with mortality in both groups, meaning that men with higher BMIs were found to have lower risk for death.[44] Essentially, these and other studies of the obesity paradox have come down on both sides of the issue. Some support the relationship between obesity and increased survival, while others refute such claims.

What are mechanisms that might explain a protective effect

from obesity? Some people believe that extra adipose tissue could provide a "metabolic reserve" during times of acute illness, or perhaps allow patients to better tolerate certain treatments. Others hypothesize that patients with overweight and obesity are identified and treated more quickly than are their normal-weight counterparts, though in my opinion this latter explanation rings hollow. If anything, patients who are overweight or obese tend to receive substandard care in health care settings because of biases against heavier people.

The distribution of fat may influence the risk of mortality even for people who have BMIs within the normal range.[45] Abdominal fat may be the real driver of heightened mortality risk because of its links to diabetes and increased cardiovascular risk. In contrast, fat stored beneath the skin may provide a safe refuge for toxic lipids, thereby improving metabolic and cardiovascular health in people with extra weight. The obesity-mortality paradox may therefore relate only to individuals with obesity who are metabolically healthy and have more subcutaneous fat than visceral fat. Anywhere from one-third to three-quarters of people classified as obese may be metabolically healthy with no initial signs of elevated blood pressure, insulin resistance, or high cholesterol, although they do develop diabetes and cardiovascular diseases with time.[46] This is a topic that obviously needs more research to be unraveled.

I believe, based on my experiences, that the obesity-mortality paradox is a consequence of greater muscle mass and cardiopulmonary fitness. Some people with elevated BMIs do not carry excess fat. Instead, their extra weight comes from muscle, which provides numerous health benefits that may protect against mortality. This may be particularly important in determining the optimum weight among older people, since elderly people have more fat and less muscle for a given BMI compared with younger people.

A CLEARER PERSPECTIVE ON OBESITY

Focusing too much on the obesity-mortality paradox, without understanding why these results might have occurred, can have dangerous implications. News coverage of the studies first documenting this relationship used them to justify being obese. Supporters of this notion argue that because obesity has been shown to protect against mortality, extra weight is acceptable and perhaps even desirable.

For me, these assertions fall flat. The argument ignores all the serious and potentially fatal diseases that are definitively related to obesity. Equating obesity with longevity justifies an avoidance of obesity treatment that can contribute to worse health outcomes. That's a dangerous takeaway. As we'll see in the next chapter, people who are obese and lose even 5 percent of their body weight experience significant health improvements. For optimal health, we must continue to treat obesity.

Put simply, having a low BMI does not guarantee good health, just as having a high BMI does not guarantee poor health. A person's optimal weight is likely to depend on age, sex, genetics, preexisting diseases, and other factors. To resolve the obesity-mortality paradox, we will need accurate, practical, and affordable tools to assess how various physiological elements relate to the risk of mortality. We also need to understand a lot more about how obesity causes particular diseases and how it might be protective in certain circumstances.

Despite the need for more information, I believe, based on the current evidence, that lifespan is generally reduced when people are too heavy, just as lifespan is generally reduced when people smoke cigarettes or contract a wasting disease. Obesity raises the risk of developing serious chronic diseases like cardiovascular disease and diabetes. It can interfere with sexual function, breathing, mobility, mood, and social interactions. Being obese is obviously not the only determinant of one's lifespan, but it increases the risk and therefore must be considered a serious health problem that needs to be better addressed within our society and around the globe.

Not every individual with obesity will develop any of the conditions I've described in this chapter. All this information is not meant to scare anyone. Rather, it's meant to demonstrate that obesity is a serious condition. Finding effective prevention and treatment strategies is therefore vital.

CHAPTER 4

What Are the Best Ways to Lose Weight?

LET'S RETURN ONE MORE TIME to Ruth and her struggle to lose weight. By the time a doctor told her that she had a BMI that placed her in the category of severe obesity, she was in her late forties and had already been diagnosed with high blood pressure, which she was taking medication to control. Ruth's blood sugar levels were increasing but were not yet in the diabetes range. Her cholesterol levels were high. Together, these factors increased her risk of cardiovascular disease.

Ruth's most immediate challenge is to lose weight. She's tried various diets throughout her life and was occasionally successful. But she always gave up on them when they became too difficult to maintain, and any weight that she lost came right back on—plus some extra. As a result, she's grown discouraged about dieting and fatalistic about being able to lose weight.

As we'll see in this chapter, a better approach for Ruth would be to focus on the *quality* of the food she eats rather than simply the *quantity*. By substituting fresh, unprocessed or minimally processed foods for the snack foods and convenience foods she has eaten her whole life, she can feel better about the foods she eats, consume fewer calories, and feel less hungry. She should also exercise more. She doesn't need to run, like she did when she was young, but she can set herself a goal of walking at least a half hour a day.

Most important, she should reconsider her goals for weight loss. It's unrealistic for Ruth to think that she can lose all her extra weight. Rather, she can set an initial goal of losing 5 percent of her weight. If she succeeds at that, she can try for 10 percent of her initial weight. Those would be major accomplishments that would improve her health and reduce her risk of obesity-related diseases.

COMPLEX TREATMENTS FOR A COMPLEX CONDITION

Extra weight is often seen as something with a direct cause and therefore a clear line of treatment. In this view, obesity is akin to a pulled hamstring, in which case recovery simply requires time and changes in activity. However, obesity is a complex condition, and its treatment is similarly complex. Successful weight loss and maintenance, just like successful rehabilitation from a serious injury, requires a comprehensive and intensive approach. There will be setbacks but the ultimate goal is to attain a healthy weight.

People can lose weight by changing their diets, increasing

their physical activity, modifying their lifestyles, taking medications, undergoing surgery, or engaging in some combination of these tactics. This chapter looks at these individual actions that people can undertake. The next chapter looks at the resources and support that are essential for success.

DIETARY CHANGES

Ideas linking food and health have been around for many years. One aphorism of the Hippocratic Corpus states that "disease which results from overeating is cured by fasting; disease following fasting, by a surfeit. So with other things, cures may be effected by opposites." Benjamin Franklin had many ideas about food and health: "Eat to live, and not live to eat." "Many dishes, many diseases." "To lengthen thy life, lessen thy meals."

Conventional wisdom says that if you want to lose weight, all you have to do is consume fewer calories than you burn. And indeed, in carefully conducted weight loss studies in which people eat controlled diets, what seems to matter for weight loss is the total calories consumed. The percentages of calories that come from fat, protein, and carbohydrates don't appear to make a big difference, at least over long periods. The fewer calories ingested, the more weight is lost.

More recent and more nuanced studies, however, suggest that the quality of food does play a role not only in the loss of weight but also in the ability to keep it off. This discussion around the composition of one's diet is not new. "Dieting" may be defined as a practice of eating certain foods in certain ways in order to lose, maintain, or increase body weight or to prevent or treat diseases. The concept of *diaita* in ancient Greece described a healthy lifestyle—physical and mental—encompassing the benefits of food, drink, and exercise.

The modern origins of what we now think of as "diets" began in the 1840s, when a Presbyterian minister named Sylvester Graham began to advocate a plain diet (along with sexual abstinence!) as the key to health and morality. In 1863, William Banting published his "Letter on Corpulence, Addressed to the Public," which became the first popular diet book. Banting described how consuming a low-carbohydrate, low-calorie diet had led to dramatic weight loss for his obesity. The Banting diet was akin to our modern-day Atkins diet, emphasizing the importance of macronutrient composition in weight control.

Fast-forward several decades, and Americans began to develop new ideas about the ideal body as well as new biases against fatter bodies. In part, this change resulted from the discoveries of how to measure food energy (in the form of the calorie) and, soon after, of macronutrients. By the 1920s, calorie counting and dieting had become a part of daily life for many American women.

Since then, America's obsession with diets and weight loss has only grown. Approximately 45 million people in the United States go on a diet each year, many at the start of the new year in response to the overconsumption that tends to occur around the holidays. Stores are full of books, magazines, dietary supplements, and exercise equipment that promise to help people lose weight. Ironically, as preeminent food culture writer Michael Pollan has pointed out, as Americans have become more and more obsessed with dieting, they've also become unhealthier. Our fixation on thinness doesn't align with our behaviors, creating psychological distress that can increase unhealthy practices.

Despite the massive number of people attempting to lose weight, fad dieting (at least in the way it is conceived in the United States) just doesn't work. The hallmark of "fad diets" is that they promise rapid unrealistic weight loss, eliminate various food groups, severely restrict calories, make unproven medical claims, and require you to buy expensive meal replacements, supplements, and other weight-loss products. In a cynical way, you can lose weight on any diet, as Mark Haub did when he lost 27 pounds on a diet composed mostly of Twinkies.[1] But the fact that you can lose weight through dieting is far divorced from the realities of losing weight, keeping it off, and being healthy. Although recent studies report that roughly one in every six Americans who have ever been overweight or obese and loses weight maintains that loss, it's not a great success rate.[2] Furthermore, a 2015 study found that not only is fad dieting ineffective; it may be a major contributor to the obesity epidemic.[3] Some kinds of dieting send signals to the body that it is starving, and it responds in drastic ways to increase consumption and restore body weight.

Thousands of "weight loss" diets purport to be the most effective, quickest, easiest, and healthiest. Just the fact that so many diets exist indicates that weight-loss efforts have been largely unsuccessful. Otherwise, everyone would diet, lose weight, keep it off, and never have to diet again. Worse still, most of these diets have little to no scientific evidence to support their claims of extraordinary results. Pinterest, Instagram, and TikTok have recently limited or even banned such advertising.

A MENU OF DIETS

A dietary plan should emphasize realistic goals and the benefits of weight management on overall health. The initial weight-loss goal that I set out for the patients I see is 5 to 7 percent of their body weight. Thus, someone weighing 200 pounds would be trying to lose 10 to 14 pounds. Studies have shown that maintenance of weight loss of more than 5 percent has many health benefits, such as reducing the risk for diabetes, hypertension, and heart disease.

The amount of weight that a person loses depends on energy intake and energy expenditure. If energy intake is consistently less than energy expenditure, weight loss will occur. However, the pattern of weight loss varies widely due to genetic factors, diet, physical activity, and differences in body composition attributed to sex or aging. At a given BMI, men tend to lose more weight than women on a similar diet because men have greater intrinsic energy expenditure. Older people have lower energy expenditure than do younger people; hence the rate of weight loss on a diet is blunted with age.

When I see patients in my clinic, I conduct a comprehensive assessment for a dietary plan that takes into consideration their weight-loss goals, age, sex, food preferences, eating habits, consumption of alcohol and other beverages, work and other lifestyle factors, physical activity, sleep pattern, social networks, preexisting diseases, and medications. A 24-hour food diary, supported with photos, provides a snapshot of a person's eating habits. In addition, the total daily energy intake can be estimated from the total energy expenditure. When a person's weight is stable, energy intake is equivalent to energy expenditure. For a woman, the total energy expenditure is calculated using the formula 10 × body weight in pounds × activity level (low = 1.3; moderate = 1.5; high = 1.7). A moderately active woman weighing 200 pounds expends 10 × 200 × 1.5 = 3,000 calories daily. Because men have greater intrinsic energy expenditures than women, a factor of 11 instead of 10 is used for the formula. A moderately active man weighing 200 pounds expends 11 × 200 × 1.5 = 3,300 calories a day. This provides an objective starting point for determining the caloric deficit needed for weight loss.

My recommendation for successful weight loss and maintenance is to focus on reducing the total daily energy intake by 500 to 1,000 calories, minimize caloric beverages and processed foods, implement portion control, self-monitor weight and physical activity, and adopt a long-term approach to health. My preferred diets are low-calorie, nutritionally balanced diets such as the Mediterranean diet and the Dietary Approaches to Stop Hypertension (DASH) diet. Both of these diets satisfy energy needs and provide adequate nutrients in the form of protein, carbohydrate, essential fatty acids, vitamins, and minerals.

A "Mediterranean diet" refers to a dietary pattern known from the olive-growing regions of southern Europe and the Middle East. It is characterized by high intake of vegetables, legumes, fruits, and whole grains; moderate intake of dairy products, mostly cheese; low intake of meat; and low to moderate intake of wine. The calorie-restricted Mediterranean diet reduces weight and lowers the risks for diabetes, cardiovascular diseases, and cancer.[4]

The DASH diet provides four to five servings of fruit daily, four to five servings of vegetables, and two to three servings of low-fat dairy. The daily fat intake is less than 25 percent. The DASH diet has been shown to lower blood pressure, reduce cardiovascular risk, and contribute to long-term weight loss.[5] Given the sociocultural and economic differences in the world, not every population can consume a traditional Mediterranean diet or a DASH diet, but such diets could be much more widely adapted to local diets when possible.

One practical approach for a healthy calorie-restricted diet is to replace a meal, such as lunch or dinner, with an affordable minimally processed packaged food with known energy and nutrient contents. Portion-controlled packages could be low-calorie meals containing 250 to 350 calories per package, balanced liquid formula diets, or frozen lunch entrées. Sugar substitutes can also help reduce calorie consumption, though by making foods sweeter they can tempt people to overeat.

MACRONUTRIENT CONTENTS

Various diets focus on specific percentages of carbohydrates, proteins, and fats, but their long-term benefits are uncertain. Examples of macronutrient-based diets are the Atkins diet (very low carbohydrate), the Zone diet (low glucose load), the Ornish diet (very low fat), and the LEARN diet (low fat). However, the optimal mix of macronutrients for longer-term weight loss or weight-loss maintenance is unknown and likely depends upon individual factors. These factors may include interactions between a person's genes and environment, the baseline level of insulin a person secretes, dietary compliance, and lifestyle factors. High-fiber carbohydrates, proteins, and fats create a sense of fullness (satiety), resulting in a reduction in total calorie intake.

Low-fat diets recommend limiting calories from dietary fat to less than 30 percent of total calories—that is, approximately 33 grams of fat per 1,000 calories in the diet (since a gram of fat contains about 9 calories). In some controlled feeding studies, loss of body fat was greater for low-fat diets. In the Women's Health Initiative Dietary Modification Trial, for example, which involved postmenopausal women 50 years or older, a decrease in fat intake and increase in fruits, vegetables, and whole grains was associated with weight loss in the first year and maintenance of lower weight over 7.5 years.[6] Weight loss was greatest in those who decreased their fat intake and increased their fruit and vegetable intake the most.

Interest in the Atkins diet and other low-carbohydrate diets is driven mainly by studies showing that the global rise in obesity is partly due to high consumption of processed carbohydrates. However, it is important to consider the type of carbohydrates being consumed—for example, snacks and drinks high in sugar or fructose—and whether a low-carbohydrate diet contains saturated or mono- and polyunsaturated fats and healthy protein, including fish, poultry, legumes, and nuts. Studies have shown that low-carbohydrate (60 to 130 grams) and very low carbohydrate (less than 60 grams) diets are more effective than low-fat diets for short-term weight loss (less than six months) but not long-term weight loss (more than twelve months).[7] Low-carbohydrate diets combined with fat and protein sources may have beneficial effects on diabetes and heart disease. Very low carbohydrate diets can be associated with negative side effects compared with low-fat diets, including constipation, diarrhea, headache, muscle cramps, rash, and foul breath.

High-protein diets have been recommended for the treatment of obesity because they are thought to induce satiety, increase muscle mass, and boost energy expenditure. However, clinical trials have not consistently demonstrated significant long-term effects of high-protein diets in weight loss.[8] Some short-term studies (12 weeks) have reported modest reductions in body weight, fat, and triglycerides on a high-protein diet compared with a standard protein diet. High-protein diets may also help improve tissue repair and weight maintenance, particularly in athletes and older people, and reduce muscle loss associated with cancer and other illnesses.

To address the long-term effects of diets balanced in macronutrients, Frank Sacks and colleagues, in 2009, published a large study in the *New England Journal of Medicine*.[9] They randomly assigned adults who were overweight to one of four calorie-restricted diets containing varying percentages of energy derived from fat, protein, and carbohydrates. The diets consisted of similar foods, and the participants received both group and individual support sessions for two years.

Among participants who completed the study, the average weight loss was similar for all diets: 14 to 15 percent of the participants in all diet groups lost 10 percent of their initial body weight. The degrees of hunger, satiety, and satisfaction were similar for all diets, and weight loss on all diets was associated with improvement in blood lipids and insulin levels. This comprehensive study demonstrates that, when considered over the long term, a calorie-reduced diet results in clinically meaningful weight loss regardless of the macronutrient composition.

CALORIE RESTRICTION
AND INTERMITTENT FASTING

————

Is there a role for "very low calorie diets" with energy levels between 200 and 800 calories per day? The rationale for very low calorie diets is to induce rapid weight loss by mobilizing energy from fat stores. A very low calorie diet may be necessary for a patient with extreme obesity to lose weight in a short time for a surgical procedure. However, the weight regain is rapid when the diet is stopped. And the side effects of very low-calorie diets include hair loss, thinning and bruising of the skin, feeling cold, and increased risk of gallstones and kidney stones.

Recently, intermittent fasting has gained popularity as a way to lose weight, perhaps because instead of restricting foods, it merely restricts the times when someone can eat. Many different fasting patterns are recommended, from one day eating to one day fasting, to 16 hours fasting with an eight-hour feeding window, to 20 hours fasting with a four-hour feeding window. Intermittent fasting encourages dieters not to count calories but rather to focus on eating fresh, whole foods and sticking to the allotted eating period.

Some studies have demonstrated the virtues of restricting the period of food consumption.[10] Although you are allowed to eat whatever you want within the "feeding window," you will probably still consume fewer calories than you typically would because you have far less time to do it. And health studies have shown positive results after fasting, including reduced blood pressure, blood lipids, and biomarkers of oxidative stress.

Many religions practice fasting during designated periods, not only as a means for spiritual growth but also to improve one's health. Although the evidence is mixed for whether religious fasting produces weight loss, health appears to improve after such periods.[11]

While intermittent fasting may work for some, it is not good for everyone. Women may experience hormonal imbalances as a result of long fasting periods. Furthermore, even though healthy foods are meant to be consumed during the feeding window, many people, starved after fasting for so long, binge later on unhealthy foods. This can result in micronutrient deficiencies, disordered eating habits, and even weight gain if unhealthy foods are consumed in excess.

In the end, the best kind of diet for someone depends on multiple factors, including age, gender, activity levels, food preferences, and whether the diet can be sustained over long periods. A healthy diet provides sufficient energy and nutrients to maintain optimum health.

THE RISKS OF FAD DIETS

If you have lost weight through dieting, you're probably familiar with the honeymoon phase in which you are on the way toward accomplishing your goal, you are feeling good, and you are convinced that your efforts are working. This period often occurs in that first three to six months of dieting, when it is possible to lose roughly 10 percent of your starting weight. However, as you move beyond this honeymoon phase and ease back on the restrictive nature of your diet, the ineffectiveness of such eating programs often becomes clear.

In general, that's the problem with fad diets, which by nature are very restrictive. Most of them can be followed for a few weeks, and maybe even a few months. But, eventually, the restrictions they involve become infeasible. We don't live in a vacuum. Eventually, you will go out for dinner or attend a family gathering that makes it impossible to follow your diet—and this will happen again and again. Maybe the first couple of times you will order a salad or bring you own meal in a Tupperware. But most people can resist temptation for only so long. And once a dietary plan has been disrupted, getting motivated to climb back on the wagon is difficult.

Ultimately, fad diets tend to work for many people for a short period. But as soon as they deviate from the diet, grow tired of it, or reach their goal weight and resume their normal eating habits, the weight comes right back on.

Another problem with fad diets is that they often fail to meet the body's nutritional requirements and can thus result in deficiencies of vitamins and minerals. People with overweight or obesity who are attempting to lose weight may be particularly vulnerable to this problem since many unknowingly suffer from micronutrient deficiencies. Beyond micronutrient deficiencies, eliminating entire food groups can wreak havoc on the body. For instance, low-fat or fat-free diets ignore the fact that the brain and nervous system need certain levels of cholesterol and other lipids to function correctly.

THE DIET INDUSTRY

Why are diets so popular if they do not work and are potentially deleterious to health? Probably the biggest reason is that the diet industry is not built to tell the truth but to make money. In fact, the diet industry may incentivize failure because that is how it creates repeat customers. In the United States dieting is a $72 billion-a-year industry, from diet pills to fad diets to diet foods to magic fixes. In 2000 alone, Americans spent $17 billion on vitamins and supplements to help with weight loss, weight maintenance, and general health. By 2016, that number had risen to $35 billion.[12] Yet a $20 billion increase in spending on food supplements coincided with the obesity epidemic.

Worse still, the diet industry and food industry are stealthily linked. For instance, Weight Watchers, created by housewife Jean Nidetch in the early 1960s, was bought by the food company Heinz in 1978, which then sold the company to the investment firm Artel in 1999 for $735 million. The American diet star Jenny Craig, who became immensely popular in the early 2000s, sold her diet and lifestyle brand to the Nestlé Corporation, which has made its fortune selling chocolate and ice cream.

Together, the diet and food industries have worked to flood

the market with low-fat, light, lean, diet, zero, low-carb, low-cal, sugar-free, and "healthy" processed food options that do not actually support weight loss. These foods are typically highly processed and tend to compensate for the loss of ingredients by adding other ingredients that are similarly unhealthy and unsatisfying. For example, processed/packaged foods often contain more sugar and salt than the original products but are marketed for weight loss "as part of a calorie-controlled diet." Often the recommended portion sizes of these products are markedly smaller, leaving consumers less satisfied and more likely to consume multiple portions.

A FOCUS ON FOOD QUALITY

In the end, the reason people struggle so much with weight loss is because it is hard—really hard. Losing weight is not impossible, but there are no shortcuts. Diet, exercise, and lifestyle modification are the best options currently available to treat most patients who are overweight or obese. And by "diet," I do not mean "dieting" and I certainly do not mean fad diets. I don't even use the word *diet* with the patients I see. Instead, we focus on nutrition. People who are overweight or obese have to restrict their calories at least to some extent. However, this should be accomplished without excessive restrictions or regulations. Instead, people must focus on the *quality* of the food they ingest while being committed to making lifelong lifestyle changes that support good health. I tell my patients that if a food does not provide you with nutritional value, it is not healthy.

Focusing on food quality requires a new mindset. When I'm meeting with a patient who is obese, telling them to eat 1,500 calories a day is not useful. Most of my patients subsist on high-calorie, low-nutrient foods. Even 1,500 calories of these types of foods will not leave them feeling satiated. A slice of pizza is maybe 300 to 400 calories, and most of us typically eat more than one slice. If you eat five slices of pizza, you have already filled your calorie quota for the day. Instead of focusing only on calories, obesity treatment must focus on a diet that is varied and filled with nutritious foods that primarily come from whole and minimally processed food sources (see "Creating Low-Energy-Density Meals" on page 102).

In general, I recommend losing weight at a moderate and sustainable pace rather than drastically cutting calories to achieve quicker results. Weight loss should be about improving health, so it only makes sense to follow the safest route to achieve this goal. When I tell patients, "Let's try to reduce calories by 500 or 1,000 per day," most of them think that's going to be tough, but it's not really. If you avoid all sodas, that's probably 150 to 500 calories out of your meals. Cut back on snacks of processed foods and lean toward healthy snacks.

Dieters have been taught the dogma that one pound of body fat equals 3,500 calories; therefore, cutting 500 calories a day is expected to decrease body weight by one pound a week, 52

Tips for Creating Low-Energy-Density Meals

For people with obesity who are struggling to control hunger while attempting to lose weight, I especially recommend consuming foods with lower energy densities. The "energy density" is the number of calories per gram of food. Because we tend to eat about the same weight of food each day, it's possible to trick the body into feeling satiated on bulkier, low-energy-density meals. Foods with a **low energy density** (less than 1.5 calories per gram) contain lots of water, fiber, and complex carbohydrates. These include fresh fruits and vegetables, low-fat soups and stews, low-fat yogurt, boiled brown rice, and baked potatoes with the skin. **Medium-energy-density** foods (1.5 to 4 calories per gram) include a wide range of foods that are necessary for a healthy balanced diet such as grilled fish, white meat, low-fat cheese, lean cuts of meat, and nuts. **High-energy-density** foods (more than 4 calories per gram) are mostly processed foods with high fat and sugar content and low water content—for example, fast-food pizzas and burgers, French fries, fruit juices, soda drinks, candy, peanuts, red meats with fat, cheese, butter, oils, and mayonnaise. High-energy-density foods are delicious but must be eaten in small portions and not often.

There are many ways to increase the levels of low- and medium-energy-dense foods in your diet:

- Add vegetables to meals to provide bulk without increasing calories. Add extra vegetables to soups, stews, and salads. Leftover vegetables are great for soups and stews.

- Eat high-fiber carbohydrates such as whole-grain bread, steel-cut oats, whole baked potatoes with the skins, and brown rice. Replace sugary beverages with water, plain tea, or coffee.
- Increase the fiber and protein content of meals with beans, peas, and lentils.
- Eat fish, other seafood, chicken or turkey breast, and lean meats (trim off excess fat). Remove the skin from poultry.
- Add plenty of water to soups to increase volume, use spices for flavor, and reduce fats.
- Use minimal amounts of oil and fats for cooking. Steam, bake, or roast foods. Use little butter spread, mayonnaise, or cream.
- Salads are good for you, but do not use too much fatty or sugary dressings! Try low-fat salad dressings, olive oil, lemon juice, or vinegar.
- Eat healthy desserts and snacks—fresh fruit, nuts, seeds, popcorn, and vegetables.

The more vegetables and fruits you consume in a meal, the fuller you are going to feel and the less you are going to eat. When patients I see tell me that they won't eat vegetables, we brainstorm alternative ways to sneak them into their diets, such as diced up into soups, substituted for noodles, or baked into casseroles. The moral is: if you focus on the quality of the foods you're eating, most of the time the quantity will adjust to an appropriate level.

pounds in a year. Unfortunately, this weight-loss formula, which was proposed by Max Wishnofsky in 1958, doesn't work for most people. It doesn't consider the dynamic changes in energy balance that occur during weight loss and the fact that some of the weight loss is water and lean mass.[13] Still, any amount of weight loss is beneficial if it can be sustained.

Recent studies have found that nuts (pecan, hazelnut, walnut) and seeds (pumpkin, sunflower, sesame), long eschewed by the dieting community for being too high in calories and fat, do not lead to weight gain. On the contrary, when eaten in moderation, they may help with weight maintenance because of their protein and fiber content, which may help people feel fuller for longer. People who eat nuts and seeds are also less likely to have heart attacks or die from heart disease than those who rarely consume them.[14] Fatty fish, such as salmon, herring, sardines, mackerel, trout, and albacore tuna—when baked, grilled, or poached—provide omega-3 fatty acids, which are healthy for your heart and brain. Avocado provides a healthy source of fats. It can be spread on sandwiches or served as guacamole.

Vegetarian diets consisting of grains, vegetables, fruits, nuts, and seeds are growing in popularity globally. Some vegetarians eat eggs, dairy products, honey, or other animal by-products that do not come from slaughtered animals. Vegan diets are stricter and do not include animal products or by-products. Both vegetarian and vegan diets provide health benefits, including reduced body weight, better glucose and lipid profiles, and lower risk of cardiovascular diseases. However, these benefits can be nullified by excessive consumption of sugary beverages, highly processed junk foods, oils, and alcohol.

Because plants do not naturally contain vitamin B12, vegetarians and vegans are at risk of developing vitamin B12 deficiency. Avoiding milk and other dairy products also predisposes vegans to calcium, phosphorus, and vitamin D deficiencies; in addition, vegans are at risk for omega-3 fatty acid deficiency, which is harmful to the brain and heart. Therefore, it's important for vegetarians and vegans to monitor and replace these essential nutrients by consuming fortified foods and taking vitamin supplements.

Shifting from an ultraprocessed diet to a minimally processed or an unprocessed diet has benefits for the planet as well as for individual health. Such a shift would support better nutrition while also supporting farmers and reducing harm to the environment. Foods that require extensive processing, packaging, and shipping rely on fossil fuels to a greater extent than natural, locally sourced foods. Processed meats like bacon, sausage, and cold cuts are particularly bad for the environment, as meat production, processing, and refrigerated transportation generate large amounts of greenhouse gas emissions. By switching to a diet characterized primarily by high-quality, plant-based foods, we can reduce our carbon footprint, helping to mitigate the hazardous effects of climate change. Another book in this series, *Can Fixing Dinner Fix the Planet?* by Jessica Fanzo, discusses this issue in detail.

Making this transition requires education and conscious effort. For example, an ultraprocessed breakfast might consist of pancakes with margarine and syrup, turkey sausage, tater tots, and cranberry juice. On the other hand, a minimally processed breakfast might consist of a poached egg, a bowl of steel-cut oats with blueberries, and a glass of milk.[15]

Unfortunately, for many, this shift remains prohibitively expensive. As I discuss in the next chapter, action by the government and by the food and beverage industry will be required to alter this power dynamic and make healthier foods more affordable and accessible.

PHYSICAL ACTIVITY

The second component of a comprehensive weight-loss plan is physical exercise. Everyone doesn't need to take up jogging, but we should all engage in some degree of lifestyle modification beyond diet alterations whether or not we are attempting to lose weight. Also, many studies have shown that staying active can help people slow down or prevent the weight gain that typically occurs as we age.[16]

Walking is the main form of exercise for most people, even though most of us generally walk less than a half hour a day. When trying to help my patients maintain weight loss, I recommend that anyone with the physical ability try to walk briskly for 30 minutes a day or at least 150 minutes a week. With the growing popularity of fitness tracking devices, people can measure their steps. A study conducted by the National Cancer Institute found that adults who walked 8,000 or 12,000 steps a day had a 51 percent and a 65 percent reduction in mortality, respectively, compared with those who walked 4,000 steps.[17] But in my opinion, focusing on the time spent engaging in purposeful exercise and enjoying the pleasure of physical activity is what matters. By walking 30 minutes a day, you could burn 200 calories, which is 200 calories that are not converted into fat.

Building muscle strength is also important for health. Studies have shown that resistance training with elastic bands is as effective as use of conventional weight machines and dumbbells for building muscular strength.[18] Given the low cost and practicality of elastic resistance training at home, I encourage my patients to use these devices to boost their muscle mass and raise metabolic rate and fitness.

However, though exercise can maintain a reduction in weight, most people cannot use exercise as the *only* vehicle for weight loss. Exercise alone simply does not burn enough calories unless you are an athlete who spends long hours training each day. Also, most people overestimate how much they exercise and underestimate how much they eat. Being off by even a few calories per day can cause a person to gain weight over the course of a year. For most people, it is easier to cut calories from their diets than it is to burn off those calories every day through intense exercise.

Exercise can protect against many of the adverse health outcomes associated with obesity, and it is critically important for maintaining weight loss. Pretty much everyone who loses and maintains weight successfully needs regular physical activity. Plus, we should all engage in and encourage each other to participate in physical activity. Exercise produces endorphins that support a sense of well-being, assists in weight loss and maintenance, and builds muscle. Even if you dislike gyms or sports, walking is all you really need to do to support a healthy body and a healthy mind.

Everyone should also focus on getting enough sleep. Sufficient sleep, about eight hours, not only protects against obesity but also improves overall health and well-being. With my patients, I recommend going to bed and getting up at the same time every day. I also advise removing electronic devices from the bedroom and avoiding screen time during the hour before bed. Avoiding large meals, caffeine, and alcohol before bedtime can promote a better night's sleep. Try to make your sleep environment quiet, comfortable, and dark.

BEHAVIORAL CHANGE

Besides dietary changes and increases in physical activity, cognitive change aimed at healthy behavior improves outcomes in weight-loss programs, and I recommend it to all my patients. For example, behavioral therapy might involve an on-site high-intensity program delivered in groups or in individual sessions by a trained provider. Coaching on healthy food, physical activity, and lifestyle change can be delivered by nurses or medical assistants working with a physician in a clinic or through telemedicine. It is crucial for participants to monitor their progress objectively through weighing, waist measurement, physical activity tracking, questionnaires on health outcomes, and laboratory assessment.

There are examples of successful weight management programs. The Penn Metabolic Medicine Program, which I founded during my tenure at the University of Pennsylvania, offers a comprehensive, patient-centered weight management approach, including nutrition, behavior therapy, medical and surgical treatment, and management of comorbid diseases.[19] Healthy Habits for Life at the Massachusetts General Hospital Weight Center is another example of a comprehensive program that includes behavioral therapy.[20] It features a 12-week group-based education and support program with a structured curriculum and frequent contact with patients. The 90-minute classes are taught by registered dietitians and cover everything from the causes of obesity to healthy eating to exposing popular diet myths. The program promotes a diet loosely based on the DASH diet and the Mediterranean diet, with a focus on vegetables, fruit, lean protein, and whole grains. At the same time, the program is highly individualized to account for a person's lifestyle and to set realistic goals.

Other comprehensive programs have similarly helped patients lose weight and improve health. For instance, on average, participants in the Diabetes Prevention Program lost 5 to 7 percent of their weight and decreased their risk of diabetes between 58 and 71 percent.[21] This program offers a structured weight-loss intervention for preventing type 2 diabetes in patients who are overweight or obese with pre-diabetes. It consists of at least 16 weeks of intensive weight management sessions based on the Centers for Disease Control and Prevention's approved curriculum, with over six months in a group-based format. The program is offered in a primary-care setting by a physician supported by nurses or other staff. It provides training in long-term dietary change, physical activity, and behavior therapy. After completing the intensive core sessions, patients receive less intensive monthly follow-up meetings to maintain at least 5 percent weight loss.

Most commercial weight-loss programs are associated with high costs, high attrition rates, and high failure rates. However, people have had some success with Weight Watchers, which offers a program focusing on a nutrition point system and self-monitoring of body weight.

MEDICATIONS

Is Ruth eligible for weight-loss medication? Yes, considering her high BMI of 41 and history of high blood pressure. Patients eligible for weight-loss medications include those with a BMI greater than 30 or a BMI of 27 to 29.9 with weight-related diseases, such as type 2 diabetes, hypertension, or dyslipidemia, who have not achieved a loss of at least 5 percent after three to six months of a comprehensive dietary and lifestyle intervention. The decision to begin weight-loss medications should be individualized and take into account the benefits and risks.

At present, two single compounds and two combination compounds are used for long-term treatment of obesity. Liraglutide is a chemically modified form of a gut hormone, glucagon-like peptide-1 (GLP-1), that is used in the treatment of diabetes and obesity in adults. Liraglutide has also been shown to reduce cardiovascular disease events in patients with diabetes and preexisting cardiovascular diseases. In patients with diabetes, liraglutide has an added benefit of reducing blood glucose. Ruth would be an ideal candidate for liraglutide treatment, considering her high BMI and elevated blood sugar levels. The common side effects of liraglutide are nausea and vomiting. Rare severe side effects include inflammation of the pancreas (pancreatitis), gallbladder disease, and kidney injury.

Semaglutide may be another promising candidate for pharmacologic obesity treatment. This drug, which helps the pancreas release the right amount of insulin when blood sugar levels are high, has been used to treat adults with type 2 diabetes, but it may also be beneficial in reducing weight. In a recent study involving almost two thousand adults who were overweight or obese, who did not have diabetes, the group that received once-weekly semaglutide injections in addition to a lifestyle intervention lost significantly more weight than the group who received only the lifestyle intervention. Furthermore, participants in the semaglutide group had a greater improvement in cardiometabolic risk factors and a greater increase in participant-reported physical functioning than those in the placebo group.

Orlistat is also an option for obesity treatment. It is given as an oral medication to block the digestion of dietary fat through inhibition of pancreatic lipases, with the undigested fat excreted in the feces. Many studies have demonstrated the long-term effectiveness of orlistat. In large studies including patients with or without diabetes, patients receiving orlistat lost about seven pounds more than a placebo group, and the weight loss was maintained for 24 to 36 months. In patients who are overweight, orlistat treatment resulted in a 6.9 percent decrease in weight compared with 4.1 percent for a placebo, and after four years the incidence of diabetes was lower in the orlistat-treated group compared with the placebo (6.2 percent versus 9 percent). Orlistat also reduces blood pressure in hypertensive patients, likely due to weight loss, and lowers the total and low-density lipoprotein cholesterol levels, likely due to fat loss in the feces. The main side effects of orlistat are abdominal growling and cramps, flatulence, fecal leakage, and oily stools. Orlistat decreases the levels of fat-soluble vitamins (A, D, E, and K) and beta-carotene;

hence, a multivitamin supplement is recommended. In rare cases, orlistat may cause kidney injury and kidney stones. Orlistat should not be taken during pregnancy or in patients with malabsorption, gall bladder diseases, or a history of calcium oxalate kidney stones.

Phentermine-topiramate is given orally as a combination medication in an extended-release form. After one year of treatment, adults with BMIs of 27 to 45 and two or more obesity-related diseases lost 8 to 10 percent of their weight compared with 1.2 percent in a placebo group. In a longer clinical trial, 56 weeks, conducted in patients with BMIs equal to or greater than 35, 45 to 67 percent of the patients treated with phentermine-topiramate lost at least 5 percent of baseline weight compared with 17 percent of placebo-treated patients. Common side effects are dry mouth, constipation, and tingling and numbness. Higher doses may cause depression, anxiety, loss of attention, and increased heart rate. Phentermine-topiramate should not be used in pregnancy or in patients with hyperthyroidism, uncontrolled hypertension, glaucoma, or kidney stones or in patients undergoing a monoamine oxidase inhibitor treatment.

A combination of bupropion (a drug used for the treatment of depression and for smoking cessation) and naltrexone (an opioid-receptor antagonist used to treat alcohol and opioid dependence) may be prescribed for obesity treatment. Compared with placebo, bupropion-naltrexone decreased body weight by 4 to 5 percent. However, only 50 percent of participants completed the study in 56 weeks. Common side effects are nausea and constipation, and other side effects include insomnia, vomiting, dizziness, dry mouth, and increased blood pressure and heart rate. The medication should not be used in cases of pregnancy, uncontrolled hypertension, seizure disorders, or eating disorders or in patients on other bupropion-containing products, being treated for chronic opioid use, with severe liver or kidney diseases, or within two weeks of taking monamine oxidase inhibitors.

Drugs that stimulate the sympathetic nervous system and depress appetite, including phentermine, diethylpropion, benzphetamine, and phendimetrazine, have been approved by the Food and Drug Administration for short-term obesity treatment (up to 12 weeks). Phentermine is the most widely prescribed in this group, though it is also a schedule IV drug with potential for abuse. The side effects are nausea, dry mouth, insomnia, nervousness, palpitation, and high blood pressure. These drugs should not be used in patients with coronary artery disease, uncontrolled hypertension, or hyperthyroidism or in patients with a history of drug abuse. I would not recommend phentermine to Ruth because she needs long-term weight reduction and maintenance.

Importantly, I would caution Ruth against using dietary supplements claiming to induce weight loss. Some of these products are laced with diuretics or stimulants. In the latter category, ephedra and ephedra alkaloids (such as ma huang) stimulate weight loss by increasing sympathetic nervous activity. Excessive amounts of caffeine have similar effects. These drugs raise major safety concerns for Ruth and other patients with a history of high blood pressure or heart diseases. Green tea, chromium, guar gum, hoodia, and gambisan have been touted for weight loss, but no objective data support their long-term efficacy.

BARIATRIC SURGERY

If a patient, such as Ruth, has tried diet, exercise, behavioral therapy, lifestyle modification, and medication and nothing works, bariatric surgery may be an option. Bariatric surgery works through restricting or limiting the absorption of nutrients by the digestive system. Each type of bariatric surgery comes with advantages and disadvantages.

The first is called gastroplasty or adjustable gastric banding. Of all the types of bariatric surgery, gastric banding is the simplest and the only one that can be reversed. Patients who undergo this procedure have an adjustable gastric band placed around the stomach, separating the esophagus from the stomach and thereby limiting how much food gets into the stomach at a time. This results in the restriction and delayed emptying of the stomach, which induces satiety. The downside of gastric banding is that people can eat very little food at one time. If they do overeat, it can feel as if they are choking on the excess, since it gets stuck in the esophagus. Adjustable gastric banding has proven to be the least effective surgical technique in producing significant and lasting weight loss. Furthermore, the bands can break, and unlike other surgical options, gastric banding appears to have little effect on ghrelin, the "hunger hormone," so people remain hungry despite the surgery.

The second technique, and currently the most popular method, is called a sleeve gastrectomy, in which the stomach is surgically narrowed to resemble a sleeve. In this surgery, three-quarters of the stomach is surgically separated and the remaining stomach portion joins with the upper intestine to form a tube (sleeve), typically about one-tenth the size of the original stomach. As a result, patients are able to eat much less than they could before surgery, resulting in significant weight loss. This procedure may help people lose an average of 90 pounds. However, it poses a risk for gastroesophageal reflux. Moreover, the reduced stomach (sleeve) can enlarge if patients are non-compliant and consume large amounts of food.

Roux-en-Y gastric bypass surgery (often simply referred to as gastric bypass surgery) is a more severe surgery that involves turning part of the stomach into a small pouch (tablespoon size) and connecting it to the small intestine. In this operation, the surgeon divides the stomach into two parts, sealing off the upper section from the lower one. The upper stomach is connected directly to the small intestine, essentially creating a shortcut for the food, while the rest of the stomach is also connected to the small intestine. That's how the surgery got the last part of its name—because the resulting intestine somewhat resembles the letter Y.

Roux-en-Y surgery limits how much food gets absorbed by the digestive system, thereby decreasing caloric absorption. Moreover, the early entry of nutrients into the small intestine elicits changes in gut hormones, which improve glucose metabolism and may signal satiety to the brain. The weight loss following gastric bypass surgery tends to be swift and dramatic, with most patients losing up to 100 pounds, half of which is typically lost in the first six months. There are improvements in diabetes, lipid levels, and mortality. However, patients are also at risk for developing micronutrient deficiencies such as iron, calcium, zinc, and vitamins that require treatment.

The fourth form of bariatric surgery, biliopancreatic diversion, is a more drastic version of gastric bypass that causes severe malabsorption. This procedure is obsolete because it puts patients at a higher risk for severe nutrient deficiency and morbidity.

In addition to the gastric band, the Food and Drug Administration has approved endoscopic weight-loss devices.[22] Gastric balloons are temporary devices placed in the stomach through an endoscope and filled with water or air to reduce the stomach space. The balloons are intended for rapid weight loss—for example, in preparation for knee replacement or other procedures. They should be removed after a time specified by the manufacturer.

A gastric emptying system consists of a tube placed in the stomach through an endoscope and a port that lies against the skin of the abdomen. The device is used to drain a portion of the stomach contents into a receptacle 20 to 30 minutes after meals. It should not be performed in patients with a history of bulimia.

WEIGHING THE
BARIATRIC SURGERY OPTION

———

Currently, strict protocols regulate who qualifies for bariatric surgery. Patients must have failed previous attempts at losing weight, they must be screened for medical and psychological morbidity, and they must be committed to a comprehensive weight-loss approach after surgery.

Patients with a BMI above 40 or those with a BMI above 35 and coexisting medical conditions are eligible for bariatric surgery. I believe that any patients with class 2 obesity (BMI between 35 to 39.9) and class 3 obesity (BMI equal to or above 40) deserve to see a surgeon so that they can discuss their options. In addition, some people with comorbidities need bariatric surgery to receive treatment. For instance, a patient with cirrhosis who needs to have a liver transplant cannot undergo the procedure if they are extremely obese. In that case, doctors may decide to perform a preceding bariatric surgery for weight loss prior to the liver transplant.

Despite the stringent restrictions on bariatric surgery, studies have consistently shown that it is more effective for losing weight than medical management.[23] Dramatic improvements in diabetes, hypertension, hyperlipidemia, and sleep apnea have also been reported after gastric bypass surgery.[24] Several studies have demonstrated that bariatric surgery increases survival, with one retrospective study showing that gastric bypass surgery reduced all-cause mortality by 40 percent.[25] Bariatric surgery is currently the most effective way to lose weight and has the highest rates of weight-loss maintenance in the long term.

These promising outcomes, coupled with advances in endoscopic surgery techniques, have led advocates of bariatric surgery to suggest a relaxation on the stringent eligibility criteria. But, in my view, unREVERSED life-long changes following surgery need to be monitored. Postoperative complications of bariatric surgery include bleeding, blood clots, leaks from the gastrointestinal system into the rest of the body, wound infections, incisional and internal hernias, stricture, and small bowel obstruction. The mortality rate associated with bariatric surgery is low (0.1 to 2 percent), but this is influenced by the experience of the surgeon and the facility.[26]

In particular, the "dumping syndrome," manifested by facial flushing, palpitations, dizziness, fatigue, and diarrhea, may occur in as many as 70 percent of gastric bypass patients. In addition, malabsorption after gastric bypass or biliopancreatic diversion can result in deficiencies of iron, calcium, folate, and vitamin B12, which require monitoring and replacement. A serious form of hypoglycemia in which excessive insulin secretion results in very low blood sugar is another worrisome complication of gastric bypass surgery. Although bariatric surgery is considered the most effective treatment of severe obesity, concerns remain about long-term weight regain, with studies reporting that more than 20 percent of patients regain weight and develop associated comorbidities.[27] This emphasizes the reality that obesity is not curable in most people and that we need to maintain nutritional and lifestyle vigilance even after bariatric surgery.

KEEPING THE WEIGHT OFF

The difficulties of maintaining weight loss have been recognized for a long time. Since 1959, research has consistently shown that 95 to 98 percent of attempts to lose weight fail and that two-thirds of dieters gain back more weight than they lost. Despite these findings, weight-loss tactics remained largely the same for the next fifty years as the majority of people remained ignorant of the effects that dieting has on the body.

This issue of keeping weight off received widespread public attention in 2016 when the *New York Times* published the article "After 'The Biggest Loser,' Their Bodies Fought to Regain Weight."[28] The article followed season eight's contestants on the popular weight-loss show "The Biggest Loser" after the filming concluded. The show, in which competitors who are obese compete to lose the most weight through extreme exercise and calorie restriction, gained huge success for the dramatic transformations that participants were able to accomplish over short periods of time. As the article noted, over the course of the season, the contestants lost an average of 127 pounds each and about 64 percent of their body fat. That season's winner, Danny Cahill, lost 239 pounds over seven months, shrinking from 430 pounds to 191 pounds.

But in the year following the conclusion of the show, Cahill gained more than 100 pounds despite his best efforts to remain physically active and stay on a low-calorie diet. Fast forward six years, and 13 of the 14 contestants from season eight of "The Biggest Loser" regained, on average, 66 percent of the weight they lost during the show. Four contestants were heavier than they were at the start of the competition. Only one contestant weighed less than her weight at the end of the show after six years.

When the show began, the contestants, though obese, had normal metabolic rates for their size, in that they were burning an adequate number of calories for people of their weight. However, by the show's end, the contestants' metabolic rates had drastically slowed, and their bodies were burning too few calories to maintain their lighter weights. Anyone who deliberately loses weight will have a slower metabolism by the end of his or her weight loss. But the surprising part of the study was that the contestants' metabolic rates, even as they gradually regained the weight that they had lost, did not fully recover over several years. In fact, their metabolic rate became even slower as their body weight continued to rise. At Cahill's weight of 295 pounds, he reported having to eat 800 fewer calories a day than a typical man of his size. Any extra calories would immediately turn into fat. Even Erinn Egbert, the only contestant who managed to weigh less six years after the show, reported that she struggled continually with her weight as her body burned 552 fewer calories a day than would be expected for someone of her size.

Slowing metabolic rate is not the only reason why weight-loss maintenance is so difficult. When your body loses weight, your leptin levels fall and hunger signals are sent to your brain. Overcoming these biological signals is incredibly difficult. As participants in "The Biggest Loser" regained the weight they had lost, their leptin levels rose, but only to about half of where they'd been when the season began. As a result, contestants continued to feel hungry even as they added on pounds.

In another study that examined five hormones related to satiety and one that signaled hunger, data showed that when people lost weight, most of the hormones involved in satiety fell while the hormone responsible for hunger rose. Clearly, the body has multiple mechanisms in place that not only complicate weight loss but severely hinder maintaining weight loss. Rudy Paul, one of contestants on "The Biggest Loser," summed it up well, "'The Biggest Loser' did change my life, but not in a way that most would think. It opened my eyes to the fact that obesity is not simply a food addiction. It is a disability of a malfunctioning metabolic syndrome."

Important lessons about keeping weight off can be drawn from the National Weight Control Registry, a database that tracks people who have successfully lost weight over the long term. Rena Wing, professor of psychiatry and human behavior at Brown University, established this registry in 1994. To be included in the registry, an individual must be 18 years or older, have lost at least 30 pounds, and have maintained that weight loss for a year or more. The registry currently includes more than 10,000 people from all 50 states, with an average weight loss of 66 pounds per person. On average, people have maintained their weight loss for more than five years.

Interestingly, the people on this registry report losing weight in many different ways. Roughly 45 percent report that they lost the weight by following various diets on their own, while 55 percent report using a structured weight-loss program. Most people tried multiple diets before one was successful. Probably the biggest common factor among the success stories was that members were highly motivated to lose weight and maintain their weight loss. Almost all—98 percent—modified their diets, with most cutting back on how much they ate in a given day. In addition, 94 percent increased their physical activity, with walking being the most reported form of exercise. After losing weight, almost all the people on the registry weighed themselves regularly, typically once a week. Registry participants also reported watching less television than the average American.

HEALTH, NOT THE IDEAL WEIGHT, IS THE GOAL

Nutrition, exercise, and lifestyle modifications are the cornerstones of weight management. Extensive evidence reveals that comprehensive programs combining dietary changes, greater physical activity, and behavioral modifications can produce an average weight loss of 5 to 10 percent of initial body weight over six months, with continued maintenance over an additional six months of treatment.[29] Weight losses of this magnitude can make a big difference.

At the same time, as a culture we must move away from our obsession with the "physical ideal." This ideal is unattainable for most and can sap the motivation from people who are obese trying to lose weight. In a study published in 2000, participants who lost 10 percent of their body weight over four months of treatment were disappointed with their results.[30] In another study that surveyed nearly 400 women about their weight-loss goals, women reported wanting to achieve, on average, a 38 percent reduction in body weight, more than three times the recommended goal.[31] Furthermore, these participants reported that a 25 percent reduction would be considered "acceptable," while a 16 percent reduction would be disappointing.

These studies highlight our often unrealistic ideas about weight loss and how they are unrelated to improved health. When many people dream of their "ideal size" they envision a weight loss up to three times larger than what a doctor like myself might recommend. For most patients, attaining and maintaining such weight loss would be extremely difficult. It's no wonder that so many people are caught in an endless cycle of losing and gaining weight.

Instead of striving for unrealistic goals, we must learn to reach for a "healthier weight" instead of an "ideal weight." An emphasis on health over aesthetics could create an environment that supports people's bodies rather than constantly degrading them in comparison to some impossible standard.

As I've noted, in my clinic, I tell my patients to initially aim for a 5 percent weight loss. Even this amount significantly reduces the risk of developing diabetes and other associated diseases. If you weigh 200 pounds and lose 5 percent of your body weight, that's shaving ten pounds off your body. It makes a big difference to your blood sugar, spine, and knees!

Once a patient manages to lose 5 percent, we aim for 10 percent, which tends to produce even more health benefits. With new patients at my clinic, we set a goal of trying to lose about 5 to 10 percent of their body weight over 6 months. The long-term goal then becomes weight maintenance.

Beyond reaching a "healthier weight," people who are obese should strive to prevent further weight gain. That may not seem like much, but in reality it's huge. Most people keep gaining weight over time. When patients show up to my clinic for follow-up visits and are frustrated because they haven't lost more weight, I tell them that they're doing great because they didn't gain any more weight!

One's weight should not be a judgment on one's self-worth or a defining element of one's self-esteem. I believe that everyone should have the opportunity to achieve their best health, but I also believe that being overweight or obese is in no way a moral failing. If you feel ashamed of your weight, I recommend seeking out like-minded people who accept your body, yourself, and your struggles. Building a supportive in-person and virtual network can create a sense of unity and relief from the daily onslaught of stigmatization. In addition, focusing on your overall health rather than your weight can reduce some of the pressure that's generated by fat shaming.

Building acceptance in the home can help create an environment that is more conducive to overall health. Stocking your fridge with nutritious foods, finding clothes that fit you and that you like, and calling out family members who comment on your weight can all create an environment that promotes general well-being. It's possible to be both healthy and overweight, just as it is possible to be unhealthy and thin. Recognizing the many aspects of health, including mental health, and giving them the attention and assistance they deserve is the goal.

Just remember, health and appearance are not the same thing. A skinny person who smokes two packs of cigarettes a day and drinks heavily is less healthy than an overweight person who exercises, eats relatively healthfully, and abstains from drugs and alcohol. Furthermore, some people drink a soda a day and live past 100 (though this is an exception rather than a rule), while others die from cancer in their 20s, despite living previously healthy lives. We are not here to judge our bodies. We must try to live our best and healthiest lives within them.

In the final accounting, the amount of weight loss should not be the primary gauge for successful obesity treatment. Instead, obesity interventions should focus on improvements in overall health over reductions in weight. Health concerns are why obesity is a problem in the first place.

BARRIERS TO OBESITY TREATMENT

Intensive, multidisciplinary weight-loss programs are the most effective option for obesity. However, many people are unable to participate in such programs. They are expensive, they take time for health care providers and patients, and they are far from universally available or accessible. Especially in disadvantaged communities, where the need is often greatest, individual change can be limited by the resources available to community members.

New technologies that complement face-to-face contact provide opportunities for intensive services to allow for greater participation in comprehensive programs. Studies have documented the potential for such web-based interventions, mobile apps, and text messaging, and this potential may increase as the technologies become more sophisticated.[32] Artificial intelligence and passive monitoring of behaviors (such as activity, caloric intake, mood, and sleep) may be able to provide feedback and spur behavioral change with greater ease and effectiveness. These technologies may also offer a chance to reduce health inequities, since most Americans have access to a cellphone.

THE POTENTIAL FOR
NEW OBESITY TREATMENTS

Being a complex condition, it is doubtful that we will ever find a "magic bullet" that "cures" obesity. Nonetheless, scientific advances will produce more effective treatments for obesity than exist today. For example, a better understanding of how obesity develops will allow us to identify populations at higher risk of weight gain and weight-related morbidity, which would facilitate more targeted and effective interventions. Similarly, better tools will enable us to predict when comorbidities are likely among populations that are overweight or obese. Given that roughly 40 percent of the US population is obese, we must develop ways to determine who is at the greatest risk for developing health problems.

Scientists are also examining whether any of the mechanisms within the body that are related to metabolism, hunger, and satiety have therapeutic potential. Some forms of monogenic obesity, such as leptin deficiency, can be reversed with hormone replacement. Perhaps common forms of obesity associated with multiple genes could have similar treatment potential once more is understood about how obesity-related genes interact among themselves and with the environment.

For instance, scientists are working to understand how hormones such as ghrelin could be manipulated to decrease hunger and assist in weight loss. In 2006, the Scripps Research Institute successfully developed a ghrelin-blocking anti-obesity vaccine that substantially slowed weight gain and reduced body fat in animals.[33] No such vaccine has yet been developed for humans, but such a medication might be developed in the future. More broadly, problems with mood regulation have been linked to "hedonic eating," as I pointed out in chapter 2. Potentially, medications could be discovered that modulate the so-called hedonic brain circuits.

Scientists are also examining obesity treatment options related to brown adipose tissue. In contrast to white adipose tissue, brown adipose tissue is an organ whose primary function is heat generation to maintain body temperature. Until recently, researchers believed that brown adipose tissue was found only in certain nonhuman animals. The discovery that human infants and adults have brown adipose tissue has sparked interest in its potential for weight loss. The amount of brown adipose tissue a person has is inversely associated with obesity, suggesting that its existence might play a role in weight maintenance.[34] In theory, therapeutically increasing the activity of brown adipose tissue in humans could increase energy expenditure. Developing such a therapy will require a better understanding of how various kinds of adipose tissue function.

Intestinal hormones provide potential targets for obesity treatment. Glucagon-like peptide-1 (GLP-1) suppresses food intake and increases insulin secretion.[35] As discussed earlier, the GLP-1 agonist liraglutide is approved for the treatment of obesity and diabetes. The peptide hormone amylin similarly has the potential to promote weight loss among individuals who are obese. Activation of the amylin receptor suppresses food intake and body weight in obese rodents and humans.[36] Furthermore, studies using the amylin agonist pramlintide, which the Food and Drug Administration has approved for the treatment of diabetes, have shown that pramlintide treatment in individuals who are obese reduces body weight and increases control over eating.[37]

The small mitochondrial uncoupler BAM15 has recently attracted interest for its potential in obesity treatment. BAM15 has been shown to decrease the body fat mass of mice without affecting food intake and muscle mass or increasing body temperature. In addition, the molecule decreases insulin resistance and has beneficial effects on oxidative stress and inflammation.[38] These findings suggest that BAM15 may hold particular promise for the treatment of nonalcoholic steatohepatitis, which is caused by inflammation and fat accumulation in the liver. In the next few years, experts expect that this condition will become the leading cause of liver transplants in the United States, further heightening the need for treatment.

Leptin also has potential in weight-loss maintenance. When people lose weight, their leptin levels plummet. In this situation, leptin replacement therapy can restore thyroid hormone levels (which are related to weight regulation), sympathetic nervous activity, and energy expenditure. Furthermore, leptin replacement can reverse declines in satiation in people who have recently lost weight.[39]

Finally, we all have different microbes in our gut that impact the ways in which we process foods. New tools have revealed the immense variety of microbes that exists within the human body and their profound effects on calorie absorption and digestion. For example, people's metabolic rates appear to differ depending on the microbes that exist within their bodies, and some microbes are only found among particular groups. These unique microbes in turn have an effect on the foods we eat. Based on the latest evidence, many modern diets high in processed foods, simple sugars, and dairy products affect the nutritional needs of microbes, in part because these processed foods are digested before they reach the gut, where microbes reside.

The discovery that the gastrointestinal tracts of humans who are obese harbor different microbes from their lean counterparts has sparked enormous speculation that manipulating gut microbes might provide a means for weight reduction. These studies are still underway, but obesity and gut microbes are undoubtedly related, and the microbial differences between people who are obese and people who are not may turn out to be important. The key is for researchers to establish cause-and-effect roles of gut microbes.

In the future, we are likely to see new discoveries that can help people lose weight and keep it off. That's an exciting prospect.

GETTING HELP FOR OBESITY

There's nothing mysterious about being overweight or obese. We know that it results from a combination of genetics and the environment. We know many of the biochemical processes involved. We know the best methods for losing weight. We also know that losing weight and keeping it off is not easy.

People may want a quick fix to lose weight—a pill they can take, a procedure they can undergo, an exercise regime they can follow—but that is not going to happen. No simple solution is going to solve all our problems. Instead, we need to change the way that obesity is both viewed and managed. And that will require not only individual action but broad and systemic change.

CHAPTER 5

How to Reverse the Obesity Crisis

PEOPLE CAN DO A LOT TO LOSE WEIGHT, but it isn't all up to them. Everyone needs help if they're going to change their diets and stay healthy. Our environment constantly shoves temptation under people's noses, and over time this urge becomes more and more difficult to resist. Without broader changes, the many challenges we face every day become impossible to overcome.

Based on today's understanding of how to treat obesity, structural and systemic actions will be the key to reducing the obesity epidemic at a population-wide level. Governments, businesses, and nonprofit organizations all need to play a role in reducing unhealthy temptations and supporting healthier choices. A single solution will never be enough. To have a widespread effect, a very wide-ranging set of policies and practices will be essential.

This is especially the case for disadvantaged populations. Limits on the affordability and accessibility of good weight-loss care leave out large numbers of people. While people in higher socioeconomic classes might be able to lose weight successfully, many others will not have the same opportunity. Without structural changes, we can't hope to make a significant difference for everyone.

We can band together to fight a system that reinforces complacency, powerlessness, and oppression. When you change your individual actions, you can influence others to do the same, which can then spread to larger systems. We all have the power to fight for our own health and for the health of others, and we all must use that power.

THE INTERSECTION OF OBESITY, COVID-19, AND SOCIAL CRISES

We are living in tumultuous times. By early 2020, the COVID-19 pandemic gripped the world's attention. To the pandemic have been added the global protests against racism and police brutality and the ever-looming threats of climate change. Each of these, by itself, represents a crisis. Unfortunately, they also intersect with and reinforce each other.

We should start with COVID-19, since it has exposed many of the weaknesses in America's health care, social, and economic systems. At the end of 2019, the first case of the novel coronavirus disease was reported in Wuhan, China. By January 2020 the first cases were being reported in the United States, and on March 11, 2020, the World Health Organization declared the coronavirus a pandemic. Two days later, the US declared COVID-19 a national emergency, and states began to enter mandatory lock-down protocols in an attempt to prevent the spread of the disease. These measures were better implemented in some places than others. By April, the United States had more coronavirus deaths than any other country in the world.

Many people have wondered why the death toll was so massive in America, when other countries were hit equally hard but have not suffered the loss of so many lives. Many factors played a role, including a flawed federal response, inadequate safety measures and social distancing, and problems in the US health care system. But as data around COVID-19 cases and deaths became more available, a troubling statistic emerged. People with obesity had a much greater risk of contracting and dying from COVID-19 than did their nonobese counterparts. In fact, obesity is one of the most important predictors of hospitalization for people with COVID-19.[1]

This should not be surprising. Obesity increases the risk of respiratory failure, alters the immune system, and increases the risk for diabetes, hypertension, and heart diseases, which can rapidly escalate in response to coronavirus infection. Furthermore, patients with obesity tend to fare much worse when placed on ventilators, with death rates much higher than among those with lower weights.

Since obesity affects far more people in America than in China, Italy, and several other countries, this may help to explain America's higher mortality rate. The higher prevalence of obesity in younger and older people in the United States may be more devastating than chronological age as far as the adverse outcomes of COVID-19 are concerned. As another example, I am a native of Ghana, where relatively few people have died from COVID-19 compared with other countries. Why are severe cases and deaths from COVID-19 rarer in some lower-income countries? A possible explanation is that these populations are younger, less overweight, and less likely to have diabetes or cardiovascular disease. Countries with higher rates of obesity, diabetes, and cardiopulmonary diseases are more vulnerable to adverse COVID-19 outcomes.

Unfortunately, the COVID-19 pandemic may accelerate the development of childhood obesity in the United States and other countries.[2] Children tend to experience unhealthy weight gain when they are out of school and eating less healthy foods. An increased reliance on ultraprocessed, calorie-dense comfort foods during quarantine or social isolation may further exacerbate this trend. Social distancing guidelines reduce the opportunity for children to engage in exercise, particularly children living in urban areas. Many playgrounds in large urban areas were closed during the pandemic, while sales of ultraprocessed comfort foods, such as cookies, potato chips, and macaroni and cheese, skyrocketed, as did television watching and online video game usage.

THE INTERSECTION OF OBESITY WITH RACISM

As many states in the United States began reopening despite surging COVID-19 cases, another momentous movement swept the nation. On May 25, 2020, George Floyd, a 46-year-old Black man, was killed in Minneapolis, Minnesota, during an arrest for allegedly using a counterfeit bill. As videos of Floyd's arrest and death circulated online, massive demonstrations began across the country and soon spread across the globe to protest police violence against Black people.

Besides facing discrimination and unjust treatment by the police, Black people are one of the groups in America most impacted by obesity. These inequities are a reflection of the health care disparities that disproportionately affect racial and ethnic minorities and of the systemic racism that affects their home and work environments. Issues that manifest through systemic inequities are particularly difficult to solve. Yet without solutions, they will continue to cause health problems and loss of life.

Black women in particular have been identified as the subgroup with the highest BMI in the United States, with four out of five Black women identified as either overweight or obese. Unfortunately, many doctors claim that this group's excess weight is the main cause of their poor health outcomes, often without a full clinical evaluation. This claim overlooks a history of racist ideas and actions that have negatively affected Black women's health. Black women must deal with the intersection of racism, sexism, and weightism on a daily basis. Body weight is only one part of a much larger burden of oppression and unequal treatment. For example, many Black women with obesity live in racially segregated, high-poverty areas, which have been shown to contribute to both disease risk and the development of obesity due to their unhealthy built environments. These complex drivers of poor health suggest that weight loss alone is not the solution. Rather, profound structural changes are needed to support health equity across racial and ethnic groups. Achieving such health equity will require major modifications of society, from transforming neighborhood environments to instituting police reforms to providing equal access and quality health care for underserved and minority groups.

Racial and ethnic minorities in the United States face multiple burdens. Besides being among those most affected by obesity, members of these groups are more susceptible to infectious diseases like COVID-19. They are more likely to be frontline workers who face the risk of infection on a daily basis. They are more likely to live in overcrowded living spaces that also increase the chance of disease spread. Minority groups also tend to be less trusting of the health care system (because of historical discrimination), and thus people may delay treatment, leading to worse outcomes.

GLOBAL WARMING AND OBESITY

Global warming, too, intersects with the obesity crisis. People with obesity tend to consume larger amounts of processed foods and beverages, and the production and transportation of those foods are major contributors to climate change. One study concluded that being obese is associated with 20 percent more greenhouse gas emissions than being a normal weight.[3]

Many people with obesity tend to lead more sedentary lifestyles, replacing physical activity with carbon-emitting, fossil fuel–powered transport or entertainment. Populations in which more than 40 percent of people are overweight have a 19 percent increase in total energy expenditure associated with adiposity.[4]

Global warming and the obesity epidemic also share several fundamental drivers.[5] Both were fueled by the global population growth and economic development that occurred over the past century. These two factors have combined to produce urban sprawl. As a result, residents have become more dependent on motor vehicles, modern agriculture, and wasteful food production systems. This sprawl has coincided with improved communication through online mobile devices, further promoting a sedentary lifestyle. Overall, the fossil fuel economy, population growth, and industrialization have profoundly influenced land use, urbanization, motorized transportation, and agricultural productivity. All have contributed both to global warming and to obesity.

The intersection between obesity and global warming places an especially heavy burden on the poor. After disasters related to global warming, such as hurricanes or floods, households with lower economic means are less able to maintain food security. Instead, people have to rely on cheap, processed foods to meet their caloric needs. These foods are often energy dense but low in nutritional value. As a result, weather disasters can promote obesity among the most vulnerable populations, which are already the populations most affected by the obesity epidemic.

CHEMICALS IN THE ENVIRONMENT

Another environmental concern is the abundance of chemicals in modern society, many of which have unknown effects on human health. Hormones in our body are disrupted by chemicals like bisphenol A (which is found in the linings of canned-food containers and in thermal paper, such as cash register receipts), the flame retardants in sofas and mattresses, the pesticide residues on our food, and the phthalates in plastics and cosmetics. Scientists worry about their deleterious, through largely unknown, effects on the body, including weight gain.

As of 2000, we were potentially exposed to 100,000 different chemicals across the globe. By 2020, this number had surged to 350,000. A particularly alarming study looked at "obesogens," or chemical compounds found to disrupt normal metabolic processes and induce obesity.[6] These obesogens can exist in cigarette smoke, polluted air, pesticides, fungicides, and flame retardants. Other potential sources of obesogens include industrial chemicals in paints, cements, fluorescent light ballast, sealants, and adhesives. Additional research is clearly needed to determine whether specific chemical compounds are triggering or contributing to the development of obesity and related diseases.

STRUCTURAL ACTION

In light of the increasing tolls of the obesity epidemic, all branches and levels of government must take responsibility and play a larger role in obesity treatment and prevention. Interventions are particularly needed in four key areas: the food and beverage industry, the built environment, schools and workplaces, and the health care system.

REFORMING FOOD ENVIRONMENTS

Recommendations for state and federal policymakers to combat the obesity epidemic include raising the prices of sugary drinks, limiting the marketing of sugary drinks to children and teenagers, requiring vending machines to offer healthier beverages, improving nutritional information on labels and restaurant menus, and supporting hospitals in establishing policies to discourage the sale of sugary drinks in their facilities. While these recommendations have yet to be universally adopted, cities and states have been taking action to promote healthier environments. Some cities have implemented so-called sin taxes to make unhealthy food choices less affordable and accessible. Philadelphia, Boulder, Berkeley, Seattle, and other cities levy taxes on sugar-sweetened beverages. These taxes have an effect. In 2016, the American Public Health Association reported that in Berkeley, the tax led to a 21 percent decrease in the consumption of sugary drinks.[7] Nonetheless, nationwide, the consumption of sugar-sweetened beverages remains high, with eight of every ten American households continuing to buy sodas and other sugary drinks each week.[8]

Taxes on sugar-sweetened beverages cannot be the sole strategy for dealing with the obesity crisis. As detailed throughout this book, the food and beverage industry is a major cause of the obesity epidemic. To reverse the obesity crisis, the government must take a more active role in regulating this industry and reducing its power over consumers.

Governments have a particular responsibility to protect children from the controlling forces of food and beverage advertising. Children are uniquely vulnerable to the persuasive nature of food marketing, and studies have shown that these advertisements directly contribute to children's preferences, their purchase requests, and parents' buying decisions.[9] Furthermore, foods advertised to children are typically high in calories, salt, sugar, and fat without much nutritional value. Through the voluntary Children's Food and Beverage Initiative that launched in 2006, Coca Cola, McDonald's, and 15 other major food and drink companies pledged to self-regulate food advertising during US television shows aimed at children under the age of 12. Good intentions notwithstanding, loopholes in the initiative decreased the impact of the companies' changes. Advertisements for unhealthy foods could still be played during prime-time shows that many children and adolescents watch. Moreover, there's no oversight to ensure that these companies comply with the guidelines and no punishments if they do not.

The government also needs to incentivize the food and beverage industry to create healthier, more nutritious products. Food subsidies could be based on the energy density of foods, or taxes could be imposed on certain ingredients or types of products. Governments do not have strict regulations against advertising a product as "healthy." Many of the food products currently marketed as "healthy" are actually highly processed and low in nutritional value. Though nutrition labels were recently updated to include useful information, such as nutritional facts for the entire package as well as for one serving portion, many people have difficulty interpreting these labels.

Local and state governments should promote policies that eliminate food deserts and food swamps. People from lower socioeconomic classes should be able to afford fresh, nutritious food while still meeting their body's caloric requirements. Positive steps include food subsidy programs, food banks, incentives for stores to stock fruits and vegetables, and zoning regulations for fast-food outlets that limit their proximity to schools. For instance, a pilot program in Massachusetts that provided an extra 30 cents to food stamp recipients for every dollar they spent on healthy food increased fruit and vegetable consumption by 26 percent.[10] Increasing the price of highly processed food through extra taxes is another strategy that could significantly curb consumption of these kinds of foods and lower the obesity rate in the United States. In our current market, healthy foods tend to be much more expensive than unhealthy foods, costing up to eight times more, calorie for calorie.[11]

While much remains to be done, the federal government has developed some programs that attempt to provide healthier food to underserved communities, including the Supplemental Nutrition Assistance Program (SNAP), the Women, Infants, and Children (WIC) Supplemental Nutrition Program, the Child and Adult Care Food Program (CACFP), and the Healthy Food Financing Initiative. Other programs specifically seek to prevent childhood obesity, such as school-based physical education, Safe Routes to School—which promotes walking and biking to and from school—and daily recess. These programs need to encourage and enable access to nutritious, whole foods that support good health.

The government heavily subsidizes the production of corn, cotton, soybeans, wheat, rice, sorghum, dairy, and livestock. These foods (and the processed foods in which they're used) are the same foods that government health experts warn are fattening and should be consumed in lesser amounts. A recent study that analyzed the daily diet of 10,308 adults found that higher consumption of calories from subsidized food commodities was associated with a greater probability of both obesity and unhealthy blood glucose levels.[12]

The federal government needs to create policies around additives and food marketing. It should not be legal to market a "cheeselike product" as cheese. A decade ago, the food industry realized that it could produce "butter" out of hydrogenated palm oil at a lower cost than butter. The food industry immediately began to market it as a "healthier alternative." Several years passed before health experts realized the detrimental effects of these hydrogenated fats.

THE BUILT ENVIRONMENT

Governmental policies that promote physical activity include planning, zoning, transportation, and infrastructure development. No one should underestimate the power of these policies. In recent decades, federal housing loans and subsidies for highways contributed to the construction of sprawling suburban developments. The resulting investment in motorized transportation has contributed to significantly decreased levels of physical activity.

Many more safe and active environments are needed in which people can exercise. Policies need to make walking and cycling safer, encourage the building of schools and shops within walking distance of neighborhoods, and improve public transportation. Lower speed limits, longer pedestrian crossing times, wider sidewalks, traffic-calming devices (such as plantings) in roadways, auto-free city zones, and protected, dedicated bicycle lanes can all encourage walking. Incentives could promote leaving the car at home or making it easier to walk, bike, or use public transit. All people should have access to parks, gyms, shops, and other destinations within walking distance. In the United States, the National Complete Streets Coalition has developed a comprehensive list of policies that local, state, and federal government can use to create safer conditions for drivers, cyclists, and pedestrians.[13]

SCHOOLS

State governments have already implemented a variety of laws, primarily in early childhood education settings, to improve access to healthy food and increase physical activity. These policies tackle such factors as breastfeeding, providing available drinking water and daily physical activity, limiting screen time, and providing meals and snacks that meet healthy eating standards. But governments need to do more with schools to reduce childhood obesity rates.

The nutritional value of subsidized school meals should be reevaluated. Most children receive at least one meal per day from school, and these meals often rely on processed and unhealthy foods. For instance, the dairy industry has a monopoly over public school meals. As a result, students often receive milk with every meal, even though milk is mostly fat and sugar. Students should receive fresh, healthy vegetables and fruits, and varied meals each day, and government should support this.

Schools, child care centers, and afterschool programs should have programs and policies that limit recreational screen time and increase physical activity. A recent survey of 55 child obesity prevention studies documented that increasing activity sessions and developing physical activity skills during the school week were some of the most promising strategies for preventing obesity.[14] In my opinion, these programs improve children's health regardless of weight, and that is the major goal.

WORKPLACES

Just as schools play a major role in children's health, workplaces play an important role in adults' health. Employers can make stairwells safer, more attractive, and easier to use than elevators, and they can post signs encouraging people to take the stairs. They can design elevators so that they access only upper floors. They can separate employee parking garages from offices so that people have to walk to and from their cars every day. They can build onsite gyms and adopt policies that encourage exercise breaks during the workday. They can compensate employees for joining gyms or offer health insurance incentives for physical activity. They can provide workers with the knowledge, skills, and support to eat a healthier diet and be more active.

Employers should focus on creating a healthier environment for *everyone*. They should avoid any programs that discriminate against people with excess weight. Employers should aim to foster a workplace environment in which everyone is treated equally, regardless of weight, while at the same time creating a culture that supports optimal health on an individualized basis.

Because many Americans get their health insurance through their employers, workplaces are also an important factor in insurance coverage. Roughly half of employers who provide health insurance do not cover anti-obesity medication.[15] Medicare should expand its coverage of programs for weight management. Insurance plans need to cover obesity treatment in all its forms.

Insurers need to create and promote prevention programs to slow the rising rates of overweight and obesity. Health insurance companies can work with communities to develop and support wide-ranging prevention efforts, such as providing healthy meals in schools, sponsoring jogging and walking events, and working to educate policymakers about how to support obesity prevention and treatment efforts.

Findings from the 2016 US Preventive Services Task Force offer a compelling reason to provide universal coverage for comprehensive, intensive behavioral treatment for obesity in children and adolescents. Even a 1 percent reduction in the number of 16- and 17-year-olds in the United States who are overweight or obese would reduce the number of adults with obesity by 52,821 in the future and increase lifetime quality-adjusted life years by 47,138 years by 2039.[16] Michelle Obama's Let's Move! campaign against childhood obesity, launched in 2010, acknowledged this need after data were released showing that 36 percent of adults and 17 percent of US children were obese.[17] That year, the Affordable Care Act extended coverage by private and public insurers of behavioral modification for obesity and of bariatric surgery. However, this coverage is limited at best, and poor reimbursement for childhood and adolescent obesity treatment continues to be a significant barrier to universal implementation of these treatments.[18] The vast majority of insurance companies and state health care programs cover only a session or two of behavioral treatment for obesity, far from the recommendations supported by the task force report. Greater advocacy for insurance reimbursement would be a step in the right direction toward comprehensive behavioral treatment.

THE HEALTH CARE SYSTEM

Finally, actions should also be taken to improve obesity treatment within the health care system itself. The way our health system is designed makes intensive lifestyle management for obesity nearly impossible. This is a major problem, since lifestyle management programs are the safest and most effective tools that we currently have to treat obesity. The American health care system practices too little preventive care and performs too many unnecessary procedures. Much of the reason that European countries can sustain universal health care is that fewer people get acutely sick and show up in emergency rooms. Universal coverage offers better opportunities for preventive care. The American health system focuses more on prescribing medications and procedures than on having meaningful long-term health services. However, to successfully maintain weight loss, patients need integrated support networks—such as physicians, nurses, dietitians, and social and community workers—to provide encouragement, advice, and accountability.

Health care facilities must also create healthy environments for patients and staff. Hospital cafeterias should be stocked with healthy choices. Fast food, sugary drinks, and similarly high-calorie, low-nutrient foods should be banned from these facilities. Health care providers should partner with communities to implement preventive programs and services directly within the community to ensure that vulnerable populations are being reached and to foster greater trust in the health care system.

Physician training and bias are serious factors in the health care system. Most physicians are not adequately trained in the nutrition and lifestyle management practices that have been shown to lead to lasting weight loss and improved health. In a study that analyzed 461 doctor-patient interactions, only 13 percent of patients received any specific diet or exercise plan, and only 5 percent received help scheduling a follow-up visit.[19] Rural areas in the United States tend to be especially devoid of high-quality treatment programs, despite being the areas that tend to have the highest rates of obesity and diabetes.

People attempting to lose weight often spend their own money to pay for dietitians, personal trainers, or behavior therapists. But many of these professionals are not well trained and are ill equipped to deal with the complex issues of overweight and obesity. A therapist can assist in the behavioral aspects related to eating, or a personal trainer can help improve physical activity, but these strategies are unlikely to be effective in isolation. Even dietitians trained to specifically address energy imbalances often fail to provide the comprehensive support and information needed to effectively lose weight and sustain weight loss.[20] For instance, in a study of 400 dietitians, less than half felt prepared to treat clients who are obese. Only one-third believed that dietitians are effective in the management of obesity.[21]

Furthermore, numerous studies have shown that most health professionals have explicit and implicit biases against patients who are obese that may compromise the treatment these patients receive. A study of 620 primary care physicians found that more than 50 percent viewed patients with obesity as awkward, unattractive, ugly, and noncompliant.[22] Physicians in this study also viewed obesity treatment as less effective than the treatment of most other chronic conditions. Less than half of the physicians felt competent in prescribing weight loss programs, and only 14 percent believed themselves to be successful in helping patients who are obese lose weight. Other health professionals similarly reported feeling professionally unprepared to treat obesity. In a study of 298 nurses, only 21.6 percent agreed that they are effective in helping clients with obesity lose weight.[23] The biases doctors have against people who are overweight or obese are often compounded by the known biases that many doctors exhibit against minority groups.

Patients who are overweight or obese are well aware of providers' negative attitudes, and this awareness may affect their adherence to prescribed treatment plans. In a study of 2,449 women who were overweight or obese, 53 percent reported receiving inappropriate comments from doctors about their weight, and doctors were identified as the second most common source of weight-based stigma among a list of more than 20 possible sources.[24] These types of interactions may also cause patients who are overweight or obese to delay or avoid essential preventive care. Reasons to avoid care include receiving disrespectful treatment or negative attitudes from providers, embarrassment about being overweight, receiving unsolicited advice to lose weight, and having gowns, exam tables, and other medical equipment that are too small to be functional.

Weight-based stigmatization in health care settings does more than just upset patients. Physicians tend to spend less time with patients with obesity, show less emotional support during appointments, and do not counsel them about engaging in a healthy lifestyle, perhaps operating from the belief that such advice will not be heeded. For example, a 2010 study by scientists at Johns Hopkins University found that the more obese a patient, the more likely a doctor was to assume that he or she was not taking medications as prescribed.[25] That assumption can keep physicians from prescribing needed medications to these patients in the belief that they will not be taken correctly.

Taking these observations together, it is clear that physicians and other health care workers should receive specific training around weight loss and weight management. Health care providers should be able to treat patients with obesity with the same degree of thoroughness and professionalism as the rest of the population. On the receiving side of health care, people with excess weight who are trying to lose weight should look for comprehensive, intensive, and multidisciplinary programs delivered by professionals who understand the complexity of their condition.

TAKING ACTION

Ending the obesity epidemic will take both individual and collective action. Neither alone is sufficient. Individuals try to lose weight and keep it off, but the system is working against them. The route to population-wide weight loss will not be through trendy, unsustainable diets. It will be through widespread, appropriate, personalized, and comprehensive approaches.

The first action we all must take, no matter our size, is to educate ourselves about obesity—and you've been doing that by reading this book. People need to understand the structural, environmental, and genetic components of obesity. They need to see the ways in which systemic factors contribute to weight gain. The idea that obesity is a choice or a matter of willpower has been thoroughly disproved. The unfortunate fact that many people still believe this actively harms efforts to reduce obesity rates.

The government should first seek to change the public perception of obesity. Obesity is largely a result of structural forces, not just individual actions. A shared awareness of its origins could foster greater support for interventions that allow people to make healthier choices.

People and institutions need to work together to make healthy foods more accessible, affordable, appetizing, and convenient than unhealthy foods. Reversing the obesity crisis will require environments that promote physical activity and social movements that encourage people to get more exercise. We need to devote more resources to preventive efforts for all ages to improve our health.

To reverse the obesity crisis, we will need an all-hands-on-deck approach. Pharmacological advances, surgery, and other treatments should complement new policies, societal practices, and population-wide interventions that promote healthier diets and decrease food consumption. Improving the nation's health may require implementing policies perceived as restricting personal freedoms that have long been granted to industries and individuals. But these policies will be essential to keeping the population healthy.

For individuals, the goal should be to reach and maintain your optimum weight, meaning the weight at which your body provides the optimal physical and mental health. This healthy weight will vary from person to person, as will the optimal composition of body fat and lean mass. Many people's optimum weight will be the weight at which they can stop or decrease their dosages of insulin and other medications for type 2 diabetes, medications for high cholesterol, or medications for high blood pressure. Optimum weight will mean different things to different people. The ultimate measure should be whether you can maintain a stable weight and whether you stay healthy.

People, institutions, health systems, and society all have important roles to play. Achieving and maintaining a healthy weight is not just an individual responsibility. We are all in this together.

Acknowledgments

A journey of a thousand miles begins with a single step.
—*African proverb*

THIS BOOK WOULD NOT HAVE BEEN POSSIBLE without the knowledge and expertise that my mentors, trainees, and colleagues shared with me over the past four decades. I am grateful for the support of Michael R. Bloomberg, Johns Hopkins University's Office of Research, and my colleagues in the Schools of Medicine, Public Health, and Nursing.

I am indebted to the patients dealing with obesity, diabetes, and other metabolic diseases, who shared valuable insights with me. They told me their stories, taught me to delve deeper into the biological and social aspects of their conditions, and provided critical guidance for my research efforts. My thanks go to the National Institutes of Health, the American Diabetes Association, the American Heart Association, and other organizations for providing generous funding over the years.

I greatly appreciate the contributions of Sarah Olson and Steve Olson for tirelessly interviewing and working with me on the manuscript, and Matthew R. McAdam and Anna Marlis Burgard for their critical editorial support.

Finally, I thank my dear family, friends, and colleagues for sharing this exciting journey of discovery and service.

Appendix

OBESITY ORGANIZATIONS AND RESOURCES

American Association of Clinical Endocrinology
https://pro.aace.com/disease-state-resources/nutrition-and-obesity/treatment
-algorithms/obesity-algorithm#/start

American Board of Obesity Medicine
https://www.abom.org/obesity-resources-for-patients/

American Diabetes Association
https://www.diabetes.org/healthy-living/weight-loss

American Heart Association
https://www.heart.org/en/healthy-living/healthy-eating/losing-weight

American Society for Metabolic and Bariatric Surgery
https://asmbs.org/patients

Endocrine Society
https://www.endocrine.org/advancing-research/scientific-statements/the
-science-of-obesity-management

National Heart, Lung and Blood Institute
https://www.nhlbi.nih.gov/health/educational/wecan/tools-resources/weight
-management.htm

National Institute for Diabetes, Digestive and Kidney Diseases
https://www.niddk.nih.gov/health-information/weight-management/adult
-overweight-obesity/treatment

The Obesity Society
https://www.obesity.org/information-for-patients/

US Department of Agriculture
https://www.nutrition.gov/topics/diet-and-health-conditions/overweight-and
-obesity

Notes

INTRODUCTION. STRUGGLING WITH OBESITY

1. Craig M. Hales, Margaret D. Carroll, Cheryl D. Fryar, and Cynthia L. Ogden. 2020. Prevalence of obesity and severe obesity among adults: United States, 2017-2018. *NCHS Data Brief no. 360.*

2. Michael Hobbs. 2018. Everything you know about obesity is wrong. *Highline,* https://highline.huffingtonpost.com/articles/en /everything-you-know-about-obesity-is-wrong.

3. Zachary J. Ward, Sara N. Bleich, Angie L. Cradock, Jessica L. Barrett, Catherine M. Giles, Chasmine Flax, Michael W. Long, and Steven L. Gortmaker. 2019. Projected U.S. state-level prevalence of adult obesity and severe obesity. *New England Journal of Medicine* 381: 2440-2450.

4. The GBD 2015 Obesity Collaborators. 2017. Health effects of overweight and obesity in 195 countries over 25 years. *New England Journal of Medicine* 377: 13-27.

5. Tamara L. Kelly, Wei-fang Yang, C.-S. Chen, Kristin Reynolds, and Jun He. 2008. Global burden of obesity in 2005 and projections to 2030. *International Journal of Obesity* 32(9): 1431-1437.

6. John Kearney. 2010. Food consumption trends and drivers. *Philosophical Transactions of the Royal Society B* 365(1554): 2793-2807.

7. Ryan K. Masters, Eric N. Reither, Daniel A. Powers, Y. Claire Yang, Andrew E. Burger, and Bruce G. Link. 2013. The impact of obesity on US mortality levels: the importance of age and cohort factors in population estimates. *American Journal of Public Health* 103(10): 1895-1901.

8. Adam Biener, John Cawley, and Chad Meyerhoefer. 2017. The high and

rising costs of obesity to the US health care system. *Journal of General Internal Medicine* 32(Suppl 1): 6–8.

9. Adam Biener, John Cawley, and Chad Meyerhoefer. 2018. The impact of obesity on medical care costs and labor market outcomes in the US. *Clinical Chemistry* 64(1): 108.

10. Yun-Hsin Claire Wang, Klim McPherson, Tim Marsh, Steven L. Gortmaker, and Martin Brown. 2011. Health and economic burden of the projected obesity trends in the USA and the UK. *The Lancet* 378(9793): 815–825.

CHAPTER 1. HOW DO PEOPLE GAIN EXCESS WEIGHT?

1. Rexford S. Ahima, Daniel Prabakaran, Christos Mantzoros, Daqing Qu, Bradford Lowell, Eleftheria Maratos-Flier, and Jeffrey S. Flier. 1996. Role of leptin in the neuroendocrine response to fasting. *Nature* 382(6588): 250–252.

2. Hermine H. M. Maes, Michael C. Neale, and Lindon J. Eaves. 1997. Genetic and environmental factors in relative body weight and human obesity. *Behavior Genetics* 27: 325–351.

CHAPTER 2. WHY ARE PEOPLE GETTING HEAVIER?

1. Larissa Galastri Baraldi, Euridice Martinez Steele, Daniela Silva Canella, and Carlos Augusto Monteiro. 2018. Consumption of ultra-processed foods and associated sociodemographic factors in the USA between 2007 and 2012: evidence from a nationally representative cross-sectional study. *BMJ Open* 8: e020574.

2. Kevin D. Hall, Alexis Ayuketah, Robert Brychta, Hongyi Cai, Thomas Cassimatis, Kong Y. Chen, Stephanie T. Chung, Elise Costa, Amber Courville, Valerie Darcey, Laura A. Fletcher, Ciaran G. Forde, Ahmed M. Gharib, Juen Guo, Rebecca Howard, Paule V. Joseph, Suzanne McGehee, Ronald Ouwerkerk, Klaudia Raisinger, Irene Rozga, Michael Stagliano, Mary Walter, Peter J. Walter, Shanna Yang, and Megan Zhou. 2019. Ultra-processed diets cause excess calorie intake and weight gain: an

inpatient randomized controlled trial of ad libitum food intake. *Cell Metabolism* 30(1): 67–77.e3.

3. Vasanti S. Malik, An Pan, Walter C. Willett, and Frank B. Hu. 2013. Sugar-sweetened beverages and weight gain in children and adults: a systematic review and meta-analysis. *American Journal of Clinical Nutrition* 98(4): 1084–1102.

4. Gayathri S. Kumar, Liping Pan, Sohyun Park, Seung Hee Lee-Kwan, Stephen Onufrak, and Heidi M. Blanck. 2014. Sugar-sweetened beverage consumption among adults—18 states, 2012. *Morbidity and Mortality Weekly Report* 63(32): 686–690.

5. Kiyah J. Duffey, Penny Gordon-Larsen, Lyn M. Steffen, David R. Jacobs, Jr., and Barry M. Popkin. 2009. Regular consumption from fast food establishments relative to other restaurants is differentially associated with metabolic outcomes in young adults. *Journal of Nutrition* 139(11): 2113–2118.

6. Mohansrinivasa Chennakesavalu and Antonio Gangemi. 2018. Exploring the relationship between the fast food environment and obesity in the US vs. abroad: a systematic review. *Journal of Obesity and Weight Loss Therapy* 8(1): 366.

7. Kimberly Morland, Ana Diez Roux, and Steve Wing. 2006. Supermarkets, other food stores, and obesity. *American Journal of Preventive Medicine* 30(4): 333–339.

8. Jennifer L. Harris, Willie Frazier, Maria Romo-Palafox, Maia Hyary, Frances Fleming Milici, Karen Haraghey, Rebecca Heller, and Svetlana Kalnova. 2017. FACTS 2017: Food industry self-regulation after 10 years: progress and opportunities to improve food advertising to children. University of Connecticut Rudd Center for Food Policy and Obesity.

9. Sara C. Folta, Jeanne P. Goldberg, Christina Economos, Rick Bell, and Rachel Meltzer. 2006. Food advertising targeted at school-age children: a content analysis. *Journal of Nutrition Education and Behavior* 38(4): 244–248.

10. Christina R. Munsell, Jennifer L. Harris, Vishnudas Sarda, and Marlene B.

Schwartz. 2015. Parents' beliefs about the healthfulness of sugary drink options: opportunities to address misperceptions. *Public Health Nutrition* 19(1): 46–54.

11. Jennifer L. Harris, Jacqueline M. Thompson, Marlene B. Schwartz, and Kelly D. Brownell. 2011. Nutrition-related claims on children's cereals: what do they mean to parents and do they influence willingness to buy? *Public Health Nutrition* 14(12): 2207–2212.

12. Ross C. Brownson, Tegan K. Boehmer, Douglas A. Luke. 2005. Declining rates of physical activity in the United States: what are the contributors? *Annual Review of Public Health* 26: 421–443.

13. Paul A. Schulte, Gregory R. Wagner, Aleck Ostry, Laura A. Blanciforti, Robert G. Cutlip, Kristine Krajnak, Michael Luster, Albert E. Munson, James P. O'Callaghan, Christine G. Parks, Petia P. Simeonova, and Diane Miller. 2007. Work, obesity, and occupational safety and health. *American Journal of Public Health* 97(3): 428–436.

14. Gina S. Lovasi, Malo A. Hutson, Monica Guerra, Kathryn M. Neckerman. 2009. Built environments and obesity in disadvantaged populations. *Epidemiological Reviews* 31: 7–20.

15. Russell Jago, Tom Baranowski, and Janice C. Baranowski. 2007. Fruit and vegetable availability: a micro environmental mediating variable? *Public Health Nutrition* 10(7): 681–689.

16. Nicole I. Larson, Dianne Neumark-Sztainer, Peter J. Hannan, and Mary Story. 2007. Family meals during adolescence are associated with higher diet quality and healthful meal patterns during adulthood. *Journal of the American Dietetic Association* 107(9): 1502–1510.

17. Cody C. Delistraty. 2014. The importance of eating together. *The Atlantic*, https://www.theatlantic.com/health/archive/2014/07the-importance-of -eating-together/374256/.

18. Jennifer Orlet Fisher and Leann L. Birch. 2002. Eating in the absence of hunger and overweight in girls from 5 to 7 y of age. *American Journal of Clinical Nutrition* 76(1): 226–231; Susan L. Johnson and Leann L. Birch.

1994. Parents' and children's adiposity and eating style. *Pediatrics* 94(5): 653–661.

19. Sheryl O. Hughes, Thomas G. Power, Jennifer Orlet Fisher, Stephen Mueller, and Theresa A. Nicklas. 2005. Revisiting a neglected construct: parenting styles in a child-feeding context. *Appetite* 44(1): 83–92.

20. Cheryl D. Fryar, Jeffery P. Hughes, Kirsten A. Herrick, and Namanjeet Ahluwalia. 2018. Fast food consumption among adults in the United States, 2013–2016. *NCHS Data Brief no. 322.*

21. Julia A. Ello-Martin, Jenny H. Ledikwe, and Barbara J. Rolls. 2005. The influence of food portion size and energy density on energy intake implications for weight management. *American Journal of Clinical Nutrition* 82 (1 Suppl): 236S–241S.

22. Barbara J. Rolls, Erin L. Morris, and Liane S. Roe. 2002. Portion size of food affects energy intake in normal-weight and overweight men and women. *American Journal of Clinical Nutrition* 76(6): 1207–1213.

23. David M. Duriancik and Courtney R. Goff. 2019. Children of single-parent households are at a higher risk of obesity: a systematic review. *Journal of Child Health Care* 23(3): 358–369.

24. Alicia A. Thorp, Neville Owen, Maike Neuhaus, and David W. Dunstan. 2011. Sedentary behaviors and subsequent health outcomes in adults: a systematic review of longitudinal studies, 1996-2011. *American Journal of Preventive Medicine* 41(2): 207–215.

25. Marianna Szabo and Brigitte Lane. 2013. Uncontrolled, repetitive eating of small amounts of food or 'grazing': development and evaluation of a new measure of atypical eating. *Behaviour Change* 30(2): 57–73.

26. Eline S. van der Valk, Mesut Savas, and Elisabeth F. C. van Rossum. 2018. Stress and obesity: are there more susceptible individuals? *Current Obesity Reports* 7(2): 193–203.

27. Karen A. Scott, Susan J. Melhorn, and Randall R. Sakai. 2012. Effects of chronic social stress on obesity. *Current Obesity Reports* 1(1): 16–25.

28. Yong Liu, Anne G. Wheaton, Daniel P. Chapman, Timothy J. Cunningham,

Hua Lu, and Janet B. Croft. 2016. Prevalence of healthy sleep duration among adults—United States, 2014. *Morbidity and Mortality Weekly Report* 65: 137–141.

29. Sanjay R. Patel, Atul Malhotra, David P. White, Daniel J. Gottlieb, and Frank B. Hu. 2006. Association between reduced sleep and weight gain in women. *American Journal of Epidemiology* 164(10): 947–954.

30. James I. Hudson, Eva Hiripi, Harrison G. Pope, Jr., and Ronald C. Kessler. 2007. The prevalence and correlates of eating disorders in the national comorbidity survey replication. *Biological Psychiatry* 61(3): 348–358.

31. Sara Ulfvebrand, Andreas Birgegård, Claes Norring, Louis Högdahl, and Yvonne von Hausswolff-Juhlin. 2015. Psychiatric comorbidity in women and men with eating disorders results from a large clinical database. *Psychiatry Research* 230(2): 294–299.

CHAPTER 3. WHAT ARE THE CONSEQUENCES OF OBESITY?

1. Ann Monroe. 2009. Shame solutions: how shame impacts school-aged children and what teachers can do to help. *Educational Forum* 73: 58–66.

2. Marlene B. Schwartz, Lenny R. Vartanian, Brian A. Nosek, and Kelly D. Brownell. 2006. The influence of one's own body weight on implicit and explicit anti-fat bias. *Obesity* 14(3): 440–447.

3. Daniel Le Grange, Sonja A. Swanson, Scott J. Crow, and Kathleen R. Merikangas. 2012. Eating disorder not otherwise specified presentation in the US population. *International Journal of Eating Disorders* 45(5): 711–718.

4. Angelina R. Sutin, Yannick Stephan, and Antonio Terracciano. 2015. Weight discrimination and risk of mortality. *Psychological Science* 26(11): 1803–1811.

5. Jenny Spahlholz, Nadja R. Baer, H.-H. König, Steffi G. Riedel-Heller, and Claudia Luck-Sikorski. 2016. Obesity and discrimination—a systematic review and meta-analysis of observational studies. *Obesity Reviews* 17(1): 43–55.

6. Rebecca M. Puhl, Joerg Luedike, and Chelsea Heuer. 2011. Weight-based victimization toward overweight adolescents: observations and reactions of peers. *Journal of School Health* 81: 696–703.

7. Rebecca M. Puhl and Chelsea A. Heuer. 2009. The stigma of obesity: a review and update. *Obesity* 17(5): 941–964.

8. Alfred Lewis, Vikram Khanna, and Shana Montrose. 2015. Employers should disband employee weight control programs. *American Journal of Managed Care* 21(2): e91–e94.

9. Floriana S. Luppino, Leonore M. de Wit, Paul F. Bouvy, Theo Stijnen, Pim Cuijpers, Brenda W. J. H. Penninx, and Frans G. Zitman. 2010. Overweight, obesity, and depression: a systematic review and meta-analysis of longitudinal studies. *Archives of General Psychiatry* 67(3): 220–229.

10. Yvonne Commodore-Mensah, Elizabeth Selvin, Jonathan Aboagye, Ruth-Alma Turkson-Ocran, Ximin Li, Cheryl Dennison Himmelfarb, Rexford S. Ahima, and Lisa A. Cooper. 2018. Hypertension, overweight/obesity, and diabetes among immigrants in the United States: an analysis of the 2010–2016 National Health Interview Survey. *BMC Public Health* 18: 773–782.

11. Yan-Hong He, Guo-Xin Jiang, Yan Yang, Hong-Er Huang, Rui Li, Xiao-Ying Li, Guang Ning, and Qi Cheng. 2009. Obesity and its associations with hypertension and type 2 diabetes among children adults age 40 years and older. *Nutrition* 25(11–12): 1143–1149.

12. Alison E. Field, Eugenie H. Coakley, Aviva Must, Jennifer L. Spadano, Nan Laird, William H. Dietz, Eric Rimm, and Graham A. Colditz. 2001. Impact of overweight on the risk of developing common chronic diseases during a 10-year period. *Archives of General Internal Medicine* 161(13): 1581–1586.

13. Daphne P. Guh, Wei Zhang, Nick Bansback, Zubin Amarsi, C. Laird Birmingham, and Aslam H. Anis. 2009. The incidence of co-morbidities related to obesity and overweight: a systematic review and meta-analysis. *BMC Public Health* 9(1): 88.

14. Charles M. Alexander, Pamela B. Landsman, and Scott M. Grundy. 2006. Metabolic syndrome and hyperglycemia: congruence and divergence. *American Journal of Cardiology* 98(7): 982–985.

15. Erica Silvestris, Giovanni de Pergola, Raffaele Rosania, and Giuseppe Loverro. 2018. Obesity as disruptor of female fertility. *Reproductive Biology and Endocrinology* 16: 22.

16. Nathalie Sermondade, Céline Faure, Léopold Fezeu, Rachel Lévy, Sébastien Czernichow, and the Obesity-Fertility Collaborative Group. 2012. Obesity and increased risk for oligozoospermia and azoospermia. *Archives of Internal Medicine* 172(5): 440–442.

17. Stefan S. Du Plessis, Stephanie Cabler, Debra A. McAlister, Edmund Sabanegh, and Ashok Agarwal. 2010. The effect of obesity on sperm disorders and male infertility. *Nature Reviews Urology* 7(3): 153–161.

18. Catherine B. Johannes, Andre B. Araujo, Henry A. Feldman, Carol Derby, Ken P. Kleinman, and John B. McKinlay. 2000. Incidence of erectile dysfunction in men 40 to 69 years old: longitudinal results from the Massachusetts male aging study. *Journal of Urology* 163(2): 460–463.

19. Erin K. Spengler and Rohit Loomba. 2015. Recommendations for diagnosis, referral for liver biopsy, and treatment of nonalcoholic fatty liver disease and nonalcoholic steatohepatitis. *Mayo Clinic Proceedings* 90(9): 1233–1246.

20. Kristina M. McLean, Frank Kee, Ian Young, and Joseph Stuart Elborn. 2008. Obesity and the lung: 1. Epidemiology. *Thorax* 63(7): 649–654.

21. Mika Kivimäki, Ritva Luukkonen, G. David Batty, Jane E. Ferrie, Jaana Pentti, Solja T. Nyberg, Martin J. Shipley, Lars Alfredsson, Eleonor I. Fransson, Marcel Goldberg, Anders Knutsson, Markku Koskenvuo, Eeva Kuosma, Maria Nordin, Sakari B. Suominen, Töres Theorell, Eero Vuoksimaa, Peter Westerholm, Hugo Westerlund, Marie Zins, Miia Kivipelto, Jussi Vahtera, Jaakko Kaprio, Archana Singh-Manoux, and Markus Jokela. 2017. Body mass index and risk of dementia: Analysis of individual-level data from 1.3 million individuals. *Alzheimer's & Dementia* 14(5): 601–609.

22. Ontefetse Ntlholang, Kevin McCarroll, Eamon Laird, Anne M. Molloy, Mary Ward, Helene McNulty, Leane Hoey, Catherine F. Hughes, J. J. Strain, Miriam Casey, and Conal Cunningham. 2018. The relationship between adiposity and cognitive function in a large community-dwelling population: data from the Trinity Ulster Department of Agriculture (TUDA) ageing cohort study. *British Journal of Nutrition* 120(5): 517–527.

23. José A. Luchsinger, Derek Cheng, Ming Xin Tang, Nicole Schupf, and Richard Mayeux. 2012. Central obesity in the elderly is related to late-onset Alzheimer Disease. *Alzheimer Disease & Associated Disorders* 26(2): 101–105.

24. Rachel A. Whitmer, Deborah Gustafson, E. Barrett-Connor, Mary N. Haan, Erica P. Gunderson, and K. Yaffe. 2008. Central obesity and increased risk of dementia more than three decades later. *Neurology* 71(14): 1057–1064.

25. Stéphanie Debette, Alexa Beiser, Udo Hoffmann, Charles DeCarli, Christopher J. O'Donnell, Joseph M. Massaro, Rhoda Au, Jayandra J. Himali, Philip A. Wolf, Caroline S. Fox, and Sudha Seshadri. 2010. Visceral fat is associated with lower brain volume in healthy middle-aged adults. *Annals of Neurology* 68(2): 136–144.

26. Daphne P. Guh, Wei Zhang, Nick Bansback, Zubin Amarsi, C. Larid Birmingham, and Aslam H. Anis. 2009. The incidence of co-morbidities related to obesity and overweight: a systematic review and meta-analysis. *BMC Public Health* 9: 88.

27. Melina Arnold, Nirmala Pandeya, Graham Byrnes, Andrew G. Renehan, Gretchen A. Stevens, Majid Ezzati, Jacques Ferlay, J. Jaime Miranda, Isabelle Romieu, Rajesh Dikshit, David Forman, and Isabelle Soerjomataram. 2015. Global burden of cancer attributable to high-body mass index in 2012: a population-based study. *Lancet Oncology* 16(1): 36–46.

28. David Whiteman and Louis Wilson. 2016. The fractions of cancer attributable to modifiable factors: a global review. *Cancer Epidemiology* 44: 203–221.

29. Jeffrey N. Katz, Kaetlyn R. Arant, and Richard F. Loeser. 2021. Diagnosis and treatment of hip and knee osteoarthritis. 2021. *JAMA* 325(6): 568–578.

30. Ananthila Anandacoomarasamy, I. Caterson, Phillip N. Sambrook, Marlene Fransen, and Lyn March. 2008. The impact of obesity on the musculoskeletal system. *International Journal of Obesity* 32: 21122.

31. Darryl D. D'Lima, Benjamin J. Fregly, Shantanu Patil, Nikolai Steklov, and Clifford W. Colwell, Jr. 2012. Knee joint forces: prediction, measurement, and significance. *Proceedings of the Institution of Mechanical Engineers, Part H* 226(2): 95–102.

32. WHO (World Health Organization). 2020. Global strategy on diet, physical activity, and health: childhood overweight and obesity, https://www.who.int/dietphysicalactivity/childhood/en/.

33. Amika Singh, Christiaan Mulder, Jos Twisk, W. van Mechelen, and Mai Chin A. Paw. 2008. Tracking of childhood overweight into adulthood: a systematic review of the literature. *Obesity Reviews* 9(5): 474–488.

34. WHO (World Health Organization). 2020. Obesity and overweight: key facts, https://www.who.int/news-room/fact-sheets/detail/obesity-and-overweight.

35. Gilad Twig, Gal Yaniv, Hagai Levine, Adi Leiba, Nehama Goldberger, Estela Derazne, Dana Ben-Ami Shor, Dorit Tzur, Arnon Afek, Ari Shamiss, Ziona Haklai, and Jeremy D. Kark. 2016. Body-Mass Index in 2.3 million adolescents and cardiovascular death in adulthood. *New England Journal of Medicine* 374: 2430–2440.

36. Sharon Hayes. 2008. Am I too fat to be a princess? Examining the effects of popular children's media on preschoolers' body image. *Electronic Theses and Dissertations, 2004–2019.* 3747.

37. Jeffrey B. Schwimmer, Tasha M. Burwinkle, and James W. Vami. 2003. Health-related quality of life of severely obese children and adolescents. *JAMA* 289(14): 1813–1819.

38. Patricia P. Chang, Chiadi E. Ndumele, Scott D. Solomon, Biykem Bozkurt, Elizabeth Selvin, Christie M. Ballantyne, and Anita Deswal. 2017. Myocardial injury, obesity, and the obesity paradox: The ARIC study. *JACC: Heart Failure* 5(1): 56–63.

39. Eric W. Holroyd, Alex Sirker, Chun Shing Kwok, Evangelos Kontopantelis, Peter F. Ludman, Mark A. De Belder, Robert Butler, James Cotton, Azfar Zaman, Mamas A. Mamas, and British Cardiovascular Intervention Society and National Institute of Cardiovascular Outcomes Research. 2017. The relationship of body mass index to percutaneous coronary intervention outcomes: does the obesity paradox exist in contemporary percutaneous coronary intervention cohorts? Insights from the British Cardiovascular Intervention Society Registry. *JACC: Cardiovascular Interventions* 10(13): 1283–1292.

40. Katherine M. Flegel, Brian K. Kit, Heather Orpana, and Barry I. Graubard. 2013. Association of all-cause mortality with overweight and obesity using standard Body Mass Index categories: a systematic review and meta-analysis. *JAMA* 309(1): 71–82.

41. Samuel H. Preston and Andrew Stokes. 2014. Obesity paradox: conditioning on disease enhances biases in estimating the mortality risks of obesity. *Epidemiology* 25(3): 454–461.

42. Katherine M. Flegel, Brian K. Kit, Heather Orpana, and Barry I. Graubard. 2013. Association of all-cause mortality with overweight and obesity using standard Body Mass Index categories: a systematic review and meta-analysis. *JAMA* 309(1): 71–82.

43. Mercedes R. Carnethon, Peter John D. De Chavez, Mary L. Biggs, Cora E. Lewis, James S. Pankow, Alain G. Bertoni, Sherita H. Golden, Kiang Liu, Kenneth J. Mukamal, Brenda Campbell-Jenkins, and Alan R. Dyer. 2012. Association of weight status with mortality in adults with incident diabetes. *JAMA* 308(20): 2085.

44. Peter Kokkinos, Jonathan Myers, Charles Faselis, Michael Doumas, Raya Kheirek, and Eric Nylen. 2012. BMI-mortality paradox and fitness in African American and Caucasian men with type 2 diabetes. *Diabetes Care* 35(5): 1021–1027.

45. Roger H. Unger and Philipp E. Scherer. 2010. Gluttony, sloth and the metabolic syndrome: a roadmap to lipotoxicity. *Trends in Endocrinology and Metabolism* 21(6): 345–352.

46. Juan Pablo Réy-Lopez, Leandro Rezende, Maria Pastor-Valero, and Beatriz H. Tess. 2014. The prevalence of metabolically healthy obesity: a systematic review and critical evaluation of the definitions used. *Obesity Reviews* 15(10).

CHAPTER 4. WHAT ARE THE BEST WAYS TO LOSE WEIGHT?

1. Madison Park. 2010. Twinkie diet helps nutrition professor lose 27 pounds. CNN, https://www.cnn.com/2010/HEALTH/11/08/twinkie.diet .professor/.

2. Jennifer L. Kraschnewski, J. Boan, J. Esposito, Nancy E. Sherwood, Erik B. Lehman, Donna K. Kephart, and Christopher N. Sciamanna. 2010. Long-term weight loss maintenance in the United States. *International Journal of Obesity* 34: 1644–1654.

3. Ann E. Macpherson-Sanchez. 2015. Integrating fundamental concepts of obesity and eating disorders: implications for the obesity epidemic. *American Journal of Public Health* 105(4): e71–e85.

4. Matthias B. Schulze, Miguel A. Martínez-González, Teresa T. Fung, Alice H. Lichtenstein, and Nita G. Forouhi. 2018. Food based dietary patterns and chronic disease prevention. *BMJ* 361: k2396.

5. Amin Salehi-Abargouei, Zahra Maghsoudi, Fatemeh Shirani, and Leila Azadbakht. 2013. Effects of Dietary Approaches to Stop Hypertension (DASH)-style diet on fatal or nonfatal cardiovascular diseases—incidence: a systematic review and meta-analysis on observational prospective studies. *Nutrition* 29(4): 611–618.

6. Barbara V. Howard, JoAnn E. Manson, Marcia L. Stefanick, Shirley A. Beresford, Gail C. Frank, Bobette Jones, Rebecca J. Rodabough, Linda Snetselaar, Cynthia Thomson, Lesley F. Tinker, Mara Z. Vitolins, and Ross Prentice. 2006. Low-fat dietary pattern and weight change over 7 years: the Women's Health Initiative Dietary Modification Trial. *JAMA* 295(1): 39–49.

7. J. S. Volek, Matthew J. Sharman, Al Gómez, D. A. Judelson, M. R. Rubin, Greig Watson, Bulent Sokmen, Ricardo Silvestre, Duncan N. French, and W. J. Kraemer. 2004. Comparison of energy-restricted very low-carbohydrate and low-fat diets on weight loss and body composition in overweight men and women. *Nutrition & Metabolism (London)* 1(1): 13.

8. Peter M. Clifton, Jennifer Keogh, and Manny Noakes. 2008. Long-term effects of a high-protein weight-loss diet. *American Journal of Clinical Nutrition* 87(1): 23–29.

9. Frank M. Sacks, George A. Bray, Vincent J. Carey, Steven R. Smith,

Donna H. Ryan, Stephen D. Anton, Katherine McManus, Catherine M. Champagne, Louise M. Bishop, Nancy Laranjo, Meryl S. Leboff, Jennifer C. Rood, Lilian de Jonge, Frank L. Greenway, Catherine M. Loria, Eva Obarzanek, and Donald A. Williamson. 2009. Comparison of weight-loss diets with different compositions of fat, protein, and carbohydrates. *New England Journal of Medicine* 360: 859–873.

10. Stephen R. Spindler. 2009. Caloric restriction: from soup to nuts. *Ageing Research Reviews* 9(3): 324–353.

11. John F. Trepanowski and Richard J. Bloomer. 2010. The impact of religious fasting on human health. *Nutrition Journal* 9(57).

12. M. Shahbandeh. 2019. U.S. sales of vitamins and nutritional supplements manufacturing 2018–2019, https://www.statista.com/statistics/235801/retail-sales-of-vitamins-and-nutritional-supplements-in-the-us/.

13. Kevin D. Hall and C. C. Chow. 2013. Why is the 3500 kcal per pound weight loss rule wrong? *International Journal of Obesity* 37(12): 1614.

14. Andrew Mente, Lawrence de Koning, Harry S. Shannon, and Sonia S. Anand. 2009. A systematic review of the evidence supporting a causal link between dietary factors and coronary heart disease. *Archives of Internal Medicine* 169(7): 659–669.

15. See, for example, https://www.nhlbi.nih.gov/health/educational/lose_wt/menuplanner.html.

16. Nicholas J. Wareham, Esther M. F. van Sluijs, and Ulf Ekelund. 2005. Physical activity and obesity prevention: a review of the current evidence. *Proceedings of the Nutrition Society* 64(2): 229–247.

17. Pedro F. Saint-Maurice, Richard P. Troiano, David R. Bassett, Jr., Barry I. Graubard, Susan A. Carlson, Eric J. Shiroma, Janet E. Fulton, and Charles E. Matthews. 2020. Association of daily step count and step intensity with mortality among US adults. *JAMA* 323(12): 1151–1160.

18. Jaqueline Santos Silva Lopes, Aryane Flauzino Machado, Jéssica Kirsch Micheletti, Aline Castilho de Almeida, Allysiê Priscila Cavina, and Carlos Marcelo Pastre. 2019. Effects of training with elastic resistance versus

conventional resistance on muscular strength: a systematic review and meta-analysis. *SAGE Open Medicine* 7.

19. More information is available at https://www.pennmedicine.org/for -patients-and-visitors/find-a-program-or-service/endocrinology -diabetes-and-metabolism/metabolic-medicine.

20. Information about the Center is available at https://www.massgeneral.org /digestive/weight-center/.

21. CDC (Centers for Disease Control and Prevention). Research behind the national DPP. National Diabetes Prevention Program, https://www.cdc .gov/diabetes/prevention/research-behind-ndpp.htm?CDC_AA_refVal =https%3A%2F%2Fwww.cdc.gov%2Fdiabetes%2Fprevention%2 Fprediabetes-type2%2Fpreventing.html.

22. Jad Farha, Shahem Abbarh, Zadid Haq, Mohamad I. Itani, Andreas Oberbach, Vivek Kumbhari, and Dilhana Badurdeen. 2020. Endobariatrics and metabolic endoscopy: can we solve the obesity epidemic with our scope? *Current Gastroenterology Reports* 22: 60.

23. Maria L. Collazo-Clavell, Matthew M. Clark, Donald E. McAlpine, and Michael D. Jensen. Assessment and preparation of patients for bariatric surgery. *Mayo Clinic Proceedings* 81(10 Suppl): S11–17.

24. John G. Kral and Erik Naslund. 2007. Surgical treatment of obesity. *Nature Clinical Practice Endocrinology & Metabolism* 3: 574–583.

25. Ted D. Adams, Richard E. Gress, Sherman C. Smith, Chad Halverson, Steven C. Simper, Wayne D. Rosamond, Michael J. LaMonte, Antoinette M. Stroup, and Steven C. Hunt. 2007. Long-term mortality after gastric bypass surgery. *New England Journal of Medicine* 353: 249–254.

26. John G. Kral and Erik Naslund. 2007. Surgical treatment of obesity. *Nature Clinical Practice Endocrinology & Metabolism* 3: 574–583.

27. Priya Sumithran, Luke A. Prendergast, Elizabeth Delbridge, Katrina Purcell, Arthur Shulkes, Adamandia Kriketos, and Joseph Proietto. 2011. Long-term persistence of hormonal adaptations to weight loss. *New England Journal of Medicine* 365: 1597–1604.

28. Gina Kolata. 2016. "After 'The Biggest Loser,' Their Bodies Fought to Regain Weight." *New York Times,* May 2.

29. Michael D. Jensen, Donna H. Ryan, Caroline M. Apovian, Jamy D. Ard, Anthony G. Comuzzie, Karen A. Donato, Frank B. Hu, Van S. Hubbard, John M. Jakicic, Robert F. Kushner, Catherine M. Loria, Barbara E. Millen, Cathy A. Nonas, F. Xavier Pi-Sunyer, Victor J. Stevens, Thomas A. Wadden, Bruce M. Wolfe, and Susan Z. Yanovski. 2014. 2013 AHA/ACC/TOS guideline for the management of overweight and obesity in adults: a report of the American College of Cardiology/American Heart Association Task Force on practice guidelines and the Obesity Society. *Circulation* 129 (25 Suppl 2): S102–138.

30. Walker S. Carlos Poston II and John P. Foreyt. 2000. Successful management of the obese patient. *American Family Physician* 61(12): 3615–3622.

31. Gary D. Foster, Thomas A. Wadden, Suzanne Phelan, D. B. Sarwer, and R. S. Sanderson. 2001. Obese patients' perceptions of treatment outcomes and the factors that influence them. *Archives of Internal Medicine* 161(17): 2133–2139.

32. Melinda J. Hutchesson, Megan E. Rollo, Rebecca A. Krukowski, Louisa J. Ells, Jessie Harvey, Philip J. Morgan, Robin Callister, Ronald C. Plotnikoff, and Clare E. Collins. 2015. eHealth interventions for the prevention and treatment of overweight and obesity in adults: a systematic review with meta-analysis. *Obesity Reviews* 16(5): 376–392.

33. Eric P. Zorrilla, Shinichi Iwasaki, Jason A. Moss, Jason Chang, Jonathan Otsuji, Koko Inoue, Michael M. Meijer, and Kim D. Janda. 2006. Vaccination against weight gain. *Proceedings of the National Academy of Sciences* 103(35): 13226–13231.

34. Maria Cristina Zingaretti, Francesca Crosta, Alessandra Vitali, Mario Guerrier, Andrea Frontini, Barbara Cannon, Jan Nedergaard, and Saverio Cinto. 2009. The presence of UCP1 demonstrates that metabolically active adipose tissue in the neck of adult humans truly represents brown adipose tissue. *The FASEB Journal* 23(9): 3113–3120.

35. Elizabeth G. Mietlicki-Baase, Pavel I. Ortinski, Laura E. Rupprecht, Diana R. Olivos, Amber Alhadeff, R. Christopher Pierce, and Matthew R. Hayes. 2013. The food intake-suppressive effects on glucagon-like peptide-1 receptor signaling in the ventral tegmental area are mediated by AMPA/kainatee receptors. *American Journal of Physiology-Endocrinology and Metabolism* 305(11): E1367–1374.

36. Christina N. Boyle, Mélanie M. Rossier, and Thomas A. Lutz. 2011. Influence of high-fat feeding, diet-induced obesity, and hyperamylinemia on the sensitivity to acute amylin. *Physiology & Behavior* 104(1): 20–28.

37. Eric Ravussin, Steven R. Smith, Julie A. Mitchell, Reshma Shringarpure, Kevin Shan, Holly Maier, Joy E. Koda, and Christian Weyer. 2009. Enhanced weight loss with pramlintide/metreleptin: an integrated neurohormonal approach to therapy. *Obesity (Silver Spring)* 17(9): 1736–1743.

38. Stephanie J. Alexopoulos, Sing-Young Chen, Amanda E. Brandon, Joseph M. Salamoun, Frances L. Byrne, Christopher J. Garcia, Martina Beretta, Ellen M. Olzomer, Divya P. Shah, Ashleigh M. Philp, Stefan R. Hargett, Robert T. Lawrence, Brendan Lee, James Sligar, Pascal Carrive, Simon P. Tucker, Andrew Philp, Carolin Lackner, Nigel Turner, Gregory J. Cooney, Webster L. Santos, and Kyle L. Hoehn. 2020. Mitochondrial uncoupler BAM15 reverses diet-induced obesity and insulin resistance in mice. *Nature Communications* 11: 2397.

39. Harry R. Kissileff, John C. Thornton, Migdalia I. Torres, Katherine Pavlovich, Laurel S. Mayer, Vamsi Kalari, Rudolph L. Leibel, and Michael Rosenbaum. 2012. Leptin reverses declines in satiation in weight-reduced obese humans. *American Journal of Clinical Nutrition* 95(2): 309–317.

CHAPTER 5. HOW TO REVERSE THE OBESITY CRISIS

1. Christopher M. Petrilli, Simon A. Jones, Jie Yang, Harish Rajagopalan, Luke F. O'Donnell, Yelena Chernyak, Katie Tobin, Robert J. Cerfolio, Fritz Francois, and Leora I. Horwitz. 2020. Factors associated with hospitalization and critical illness among 4,103 patients with COVID-19 disease in New York City. *BMJ* 369: m1966.

2. Andrew G. Rundle, Yoosun Park, Julie B. Herbstman, Eliza W. Kinsey, and Y. Claire Wang. 2020. COVID-19 related school closings and risk of weight gain among children. *Obesity* 28(6): 1008–1009.

3. Faidon Magkos, Inge Tetens, Susanne Gjedsted Bügel, Claus Felby, Simon Rønnow Schacht, James O. Hill, Eric Ravussin, and Arne Astrup. 2019. The environmental foodprint of obesity. *Obesity* 28(1): 73–79.

4. Gary Webb and Garry Egger. 2013. Obesity and climate change: can we link the two and can we deal with both together? *American Journal of Lifestyle Medicine* 8(3): 200–204.

5. Ruopeng An, Mengmeng Ji, and Shuying Zhang. 2017. Global warming and obesity: a systematic review. *Obesity Reviews* 19: 150–163.

6. Marco E. Franco, Maria T. Fernandex-Luna, Alejandro J. Ramirez, and Ramon Lavado. 2020. Metabolic-based assessment reveals dysregulation of lipid profiles in human liver cells exposed to environmental obesogens. *Toxicology and Applied Pharmacology* 398: 11509.

7. Jennifer Falbe, Hannah R. Thompson, Christina M. Becker, Nadia Rojas, Charles E. McCulloch, and Kristine A. Madsen. 2016. The impact of the Berkeley Excise Tax on sugar-sweetened beverage consumption. *American Journal of Public Health* 106(10): 1865–1871.

8. E. J. Mundell. 2019. Sugar sodas still popular, but warnings, taxes can curb uptake *U.S. News and World Report,* https://www.usnews.com/news/health-news/articles/2019-06-09/sugary-sodas-still-popular-but-warnings-taxes-can-curb-uptake.

9. Institute of Medicine. 2006. *Food Marketing to Children and Youth: Threat or Opportunity?* Washington, DC: National Academies Press.

10. Susan Bartlett, Jacob Klerman, Lauren Olsho, Christopher Logan, Michelle Blocklin, Marianne Beauregard, Ayesha Enver, Park Wilde, Cheryl Owens, and Margaret Melhem. 2014. *Evaluation of the Healthy Incentives Pilot (HIP): Final Report.* Prepared by Abt Associates for the Food and Nutrition Service of the US Department of Agriculture.

11. Pablo Monsivais, Julia Mclain, and Adam Drewnowski. 2010. The rising disparity in the price of healthful foods: 2004–2008. *Food Policy* 35(6): 514–520.

12. Karen R. Siegel, Kai McKeever Bullard, Giuseppina Imperatore, Henry S. Kahn, Aryeh D. Stein, Mohammed K. Ali, and K. M. Narayan. 2016. Association of higher consumption of foods derived from subsidized commodities with adverse cardiometabolic risk among US adults. *JAMA Internal Medicine* 176(8): 1124–1132.

13. More information is available at the website of Smart Growth America, https://smartgrowthamerica.org/program/national-complete-streets -coalition/.

14. Tamara Brown, Theresa Hm Moore, Lee Hooper, Yang Gao, Amir Zayegh, Sharea Ijaz, Martha Elwenspoek, Sophie C. Foxen, Lucia Magee, Claire O'Malley, Elizabeth Waters, and Carolyn D. Summerbell. 2019. Interventions for preventing obesity in children. *Cochrane Database of Systemic Reviews* 7(7): CD001871.

15. National Academies of Sciences, Engineering, and Medicine. 2017. *The challenge of treating obesity and overweight: Proceedings of a workshop.* Washington, DC: National Academies Press.

16. Li Y. Yang, Maxine Denniston, Sarah Lee, Deborah Galuska, and Richard Lowry. 2010. Long-term health and economic impact of preventing and reducing overweight and obesity in adolescence. *Journal of Adolescent Health* 46(5): 467–473.

17. Cynthia L. Ogden, Margaret D. Carroll, Brian K. Kit, and Katherine M. Flegal. 2012. Prevalence of obesity in the United States, 2009–2010. *NCHS Data Brief* 82: 1–8.

18. Wendy Slusser, Karan Staten, Karen Stephens, Lenna Liu, Christine Yeh, Sarah Armstrong, Daniel A. DeUgarte, and Matthew Haemer. 2011. Payment for obesity services: examples and recommendations for stage 3 comprehensive multidisciplinary intervention programs for children and adolescents. *Pediatrics* 128 (Suppl 2): S78–S85.

19. Stewart C. Alexander, Mary E. Coz, Christy L. Boling Turer, Pauline Lyne, Truls Ostbye, James A. Tulsky, Rowena J. Dolor, and Kathryn I. Pollak. 2011. Do the five A's work when physicians counsel about weight loss. *Family Medicine* 43(3): 179–184.

20. Karen Jane Campbell and D. Crawford. 2000. Management of obesity: attitudes and practices of Australian dietitians. *International Journal of Obesity* 24(6): 701–710.

21. Thomas A. Wadden, Drew A. Anderson, Gary D. Foster, A. Bennett, C. Steinberg, and D. B. Sarwer. 2000. Obese women's perceptions of their physicians' weight management attitudes and practices. *Archives of Family Medicine* 9(9): 854–860.

22. Gary D. Foster, Thomas A. Wadden, Angela P. Makris, Duncan Davidson, Rebecca Swain Sanderson, David B. Allison, and Amy Kessler. 2012. Primary care physicians' attitudes about obesity and its treatment. *Obesity* 11(10): 1168–1177.

23. Ian Brown, Chris Stride, Alkaterini Psarou, Louise Brewins, and Joanne Thompson. 2007. Management of obesity in primary care: nurses' practices, beliefs, and attitudes. *Journal of Advanced Nursing* 59(4): 329–341.

24. Rebecca M. Puhl and Kelly D. Brownell. 2006. Confronting and coping with weight stigma: an investigation of overweight and obese adults. *Obesity* 14(10): 1802–1815.

25. Sharon Begley. 2012. Insight: America's hatred of fat hurts obesity fight. *Reuters,* https://www.reuters.com/article/us-obesity-stigma/insight -americas-hatred-of-fat-hurts-obesity-fight-idUSBRE84A0PA20120511.

Index

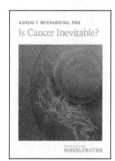
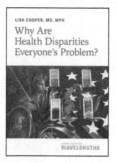
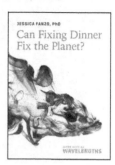
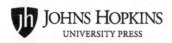